Edited by
HUGH FREEMAN
JOHN HENDERSON

Evaluation of Comprehensive Care of the Mentally Ill

The Transition from Mental Hospital
Care to Extramural Care of the Mentally
Ill in European Community Countries

GASKELL

©The Royal College of Psychiatrists 1991

ISBN 0 902241 39 7

Gaskell is an imprint of the Royal College of Psychiatrists,
17 Belgrave Square, London SW1

Distributed in North America
by American Psychiatric Press, Inc.
ISBN 0 88048 606 6

British Library Cataloguing in Publication Data
Evaluation of comprehensive care of the mentally ill:
the transition from mental hospital care to
extramural care of the mentally ill in European
Community countries.
I. Title
610.7368094

ISBN 0-902241-39-7

Phototypeset by Dobbie Typesetting Limited, Tavistock, Devon
Printed in Great Britain by Bell and Bain Ltd., Glasgow

Evaluation of Comprehensive Care of the Mentally Ill

Contents

List of contributors   vii
Foreword   *Michael Shepherd*   ix
Introduction   *Hugh Freeman and John H. Henderson*   xi

1   Methodology of evaluative studies in the mental health field
    Heinz Häfner and Wolfram an der Heiden   1
    Discussion   *John K. Wing*   18
2   Effectiveness of treatment strategies for the chronic mentally ill
    Marianne Kastrup   24
3   The establishment, monitoring and evaluation of community
    care services   *C. L. Cazzullo, G. Tacchini, Carlo Altamura
    and Michele Tansella*   30
4   Services for patients with chronic mental illness: results of research
    and experience   *John Shanks*   45
    Discussion   *Nikolas Manos*   53
5   Effectiveness of the wider social network in community care of
    the mentally ill   *Joris Casselman*   57
    Discussion   *Roger Amiel*   65
6   Evaluation of change in the system of mental health care
    Durk Wiersma and Robert Giel   68
7   Do long-stay patients benefit from community placement?
    J. P. Leff   79
    Discussion   *Raimo K. R. Salokangas*   91
8   Improving the social competence of the chronic mentally ill
    Hans D. Brenner, Milka Maurer and Marco C. G. Merlo   97
9   Integrating mental health in primary health care
    David Goldberg   115
    Discussion   *Tom Fahy*   125

10 Process or outcome approach in the evaluation of psychiatric
    services   *Pierluigi Morosini and Franco Veltro*   127
11 The direct costs of the community care of chronic mentally
    ill people   *Martin Knapp*   142
12 Cost-effectiveness of community care for the chronic mentally
    ill   *Owen O'Donnell*   174
13 National reports
    France: *Roger Amiel*   197
    Greece: *Nicolas Zachariadis*   198
    The Netherlands: *Durk Wiersma*   198
    Portugal: *José Caldas de Almeido*   199
    Spain: *Carlos Artundo Purroy*   201

Contributors

Carlo Altamura, Istituto di Clinica Psichiatrica, Guardia II, Ospedale Maggiore, Milan, Italy

Roger Amiel, Psychiatre des Hôpitaux, Paris, France

Wolfram an der Heiden, Zentralinstitut für Seelische Gesundheit, Mannheim, Germany

Carlos Artundo Purroy, c/Ciudadela 5, 31001 Pamplona, Spain

Hans D. Brenner, Psychiatrische Universitätsklinik Bern, Abteilung für Theoretische und Evaluative Psychiatrie, Bern, Switzerland

José Caldas de Almeida, Clinica Universitária de Saúde Mental e Psiquitaria, Lisbon, Portugal

Joris Casselman, Katholieke Universiteit Leuven, Universitair Psychiatrisch Centrum, Bierbeek, Belgium

C. L. Cazzullo, Department of Psychiatry, University of Milan, Milan, Italy

Tom Fahy, Department of Psychiatry, University College Hospital, Galway, Ireland

Hugh Freeman, Editor, *British Journal of Psychiatry*, London, UK

Robert Giel, Department of Social Psychiatry, University of Groningen, Groningen, the Netherlands

David Goldberg, Mental Illness Research Unit, Withington Hospital and University of Manchester, Manchester, UK

Heinz Häfner, Zentralinstitut für Seelische Gesundheit, Mannheim, Germany

John H. Henderson, St. Andrew's Hospital, Northampton, UK

Marianne Kastrup, Psychiatric Department, Hvidovre Hospital, Hvidovre, Denmark

Martin Knapp, Personal Social Services Research Unit, University of Kent at Canterbury, Canterbury, UK

Julian Leff, Director, MRC Social Psychiatry Unit, Friern Hospital, London, UK

Nikolas Manos, Community Mental Health Centre, Thessaloníki, Greece

Milka Maurer, Psychiatrische Universitätsklinik Bern, Abteilung für Theoretische und Evaluative Psychiatrie, Bern, Switzerland

Marco C. G. Merlo, Psychiatrische Universitätsklinik Bern, Abteilung für Theoretische und Evaluative Psychiatrie, Bern, Switzerland

Pierluigi Morosini, Laboratorio di Epidemiologia e Biostatistica, Istituto Superiore di Sanita, Rome, Italy

Owen O'Donnell, Centre for Health Economics, University of York, York, UK

Raimo K. R. Salokangas, Department of Public Health, University of Tampere, Tampere, Finland

John Shanks, Principal Medical Officer, Department of Health, Wellington House, London, UK

Michael Shepherd, Institute of Psychiatry, De Crespigny Park, London, UK

G. Tacchini, Istituto di Clinica Psichiatrica, Guardia II, Ospedale Maggiore, Milan, Italy

Michele Tansella, Istituto di Psichiatria, Università di Verona, Verona, Italy

Franco Veltro, Laboratorio di Epidemiologia e Biostatistica, Istituto Superiore di Sanita, Rome, Italy

Durk Wiersma, Department of Social Psychiatry, University of Groningen, Groningen, the Netherlands

John K. Wing, Research Unit, Royal College of Psychiatrists, London, UK

Nicolas A. Zachariadis, Director of Psychiatric Unit, Psychiatric Hospital of Attica, Athens, Greece

Foreword

MICHAEL SHEPHERD

In his book *Mental Health Care in the European Community* (1985), Steen Mangen provided a comparative account of the developments and constraints of the policies adopted by the nine full-member states of the European Community (EC) from the 1960s to the early 1980s. The contributors presented several variations on the common theme of a movement from institutional to community care in the light of national differences in health care systems, changing social attitudes, and economic limitations. From the descriptions, it was apparent that each country had proceeded in its own way and that there had been very little in the way of collaboration, despite the existence of three European organisations which are potentially well placed for such activity. However, as Mangen pointed out, the roles of two of these bodies – the Council of Europe and the World Health Organization – are "advisory and exhortative". Of the third, the Commission of the European Communities (CEC), he commented that "no attempt is currently being made to seek an integration of the diverse health care systems of EC countries. Nor is such harmonisation likely in the future, since it is improbable that national governments will be willing to surrender responsibilities in areas of social policy such as health care which consume significant proportions of their GNP (p. 267)".

Despite this pessimistic pronouncement, it was in the same year as the appearance of Mangen's volume that European Health Ministers provided an initiative which led to the formation of a planning group to examine some aspects of mental health care in EC member states, with particular reference to the need for evaluating the issues raised by the transition from hospital to extramural care (see the editors' Introduction). As a preliminary measure, the planning group, after considering several possibilities, decided to organise a workshop at which representatives of 12 countries were invited to take a broad, multifaceted view of the current situation: their papers and those of invited discussants make up the core of the proceedings reported in this volume. In addition, there are brief reports on the status quo in each of the individual countries as this relates to the administrative background, the delivery of specialised care, the role of primary health services, and the place of private practice, and charitable and voluntary organisations in the provision of psychiatric services.

On the foundations of this information, it is proposed to mount a CEC-concerted action programme on the delivery of mental health services, through the setting up of coordinated field studies, designed to evaluate the relative medical, social, and economic advantages and disadvantages of care in hospital and in the community, respectively. Sound epidemiological research of this type should help fill many gaps in knowledge, and furnish a factual underpinning for clinical management as well as for policy decisions. It is not always appreciated that in psychiatry, as in other branches of medicine, "the medical profession has had very little say in the major decisions about the design of the health services" (Cooper, 1990, pp. 251–252). This historical observation may be contrasted with the now widely accepted tenet that "the discipline of epidemiology should be a major pillar in the formulation and implementation of health policy" (Levine & Lilienfeld, 1987). To this end, the acquisition of relevant data constitutes an indispensable first step. It is to be hoped that from the material assembled in this valuable compilation, will emerge the guidelines needed for a rational mental health programme in the European Community.

References

COOPER, J. E. (1990) Professional obstacles to implementation and diffusion of innovative approaches to mental health care. In *Mental Health Care Delivery: Innovations, Impediments and Implementation* (eds I. M. Marks & R. A. Scott), pp. 251–252. Cambridge: Cambridge University Press.

LEVINE, S. & LILIENFELD, A. (eds) (1987) *Epidemiology and Health Policy*. London: Tavistock.

MANGEN, S. P. (ed.) (1985) *Mental Health in the European Community*. London: Croom Helm.

Introduction

HUGH FREEMAN and JOHN H. HENDERSON

At the Second Conference of European Health Ministers convened by the Council of Europe (CE) and held in Stockholm, Sweden, in April 1985, the Ministers of Health, or their representatives, from 21 member states, reaffirmed the importance of mental health promotion and of the prevention and treatment of mental disorders as essential components of a comprehensive health policy. The Conference revealed a unity of commitment by Ministers to a number of common principles of policy, practice, and implementation of comprehensive community-based mental health care. The final text of the Conference, adopted at the conclusion of the meeting, contained a number of such matters of policy and practice on which firm agreement was reached. These composed a foundation for a European strategy for the promotion of mental health and for the development of community-based, diversified programmes for the treatment, rehabilitation, and prevention of mental disorders (Ref: CM(85)117 Council of Europe).

In July 1985, the Commission of the European Communities (CEC) Programme on Medical and Health Research invited interested researchers on mental health care within the European Community member states (EC) to undertake the planning of a workshop and an intercountry collaborative study of evaluation of the transition from traditional mental hospital to extramural community care of mentally ill patients, in the EC member states. The group, which was established by the Concerted Action Committee Health Service Research (COMAC-HSR) of the CEC, was invited to consider the need for a collaborative approach among member states to study and investigate the ongoing process of deinstitutionalisation of patients from mental health care. In particular, the group was required to consider the interest shown by EC member states in the rapidity of this change in policy towards community-based care, to consider the social importance of these changes, and to examine the economic importance of the changes in practice.

The work of the planning group was governed by its principal aim. This was to furnish policy makers, health administrators, and clinical decision-makers with sufficient information from evaluation research on mental health care to encourage, enhance, and ensure a smooth transition from traditional institutional mental care to a comprehensive, community-based, and diversified service for the treatment, rehabilitation, and prevention of mental disorders. From July 1985 to October 1986, this planning group met on four occasions. It was charged with the task of formulating proposals to investigate and evaluate the outcome of the transition from traditional mental hospital care of the mentally ill towards extramural care, in EC member states.

The first activity undertaken was a workshop held in London in December 1989, the proceedings of which make up the contents of this publication. For this workshop, the programme chosen was focused on presentations of recent evaluation studies of a selection of local and national experiences of developing alternatives to traditional mental hospital care. It was considered important to also include papers and discussion on methodology of evaluation studies in mental health care delivery systems, studies of the effectiveness of treatment strategies for the chronic mentally ill patient, and methods to improve the social competence of such patients.

The two-year outcome study of a long-term assessment of a mental hospital closure programme gives an account of both the methods and outcome of community placement programmes. Cost-effectiveness studies of mental health policy changes and implementation are introduced, and examples included of direct costing projects on community placement of the chronic mentally ill patient.

Given that, in Europe, the trend towards deinstitutionalisation has reached its greatest momentum in Italy, two studies of community care in northern Italy are described. A secondary, but nevertheless important and inescapable, contribution to changing policies in health care and their impact on mental health care is the worldwide commitment to primary health care as the basis of the WHO movement to Health for All. Mental health care delivery is influenced significantly by primary health care developments, and a review of these is included in the proceedings.

In the discussions which were centred on each working paper, frequent reference was made to the experiences of individual countries in coping with the movement to transfer mental health care and treatment from mental hospitals to alternatives in the community. There was agreement that the movement was taking place discernibly in every country, although each one was at a different stage of the transition, and within each country, there were noticeably different local patterns of change in policy and practice.

Nevertheless, a steady decline in the number of resident chronic patients has resulted in most countries, a fact which has reinforced the predominant theme of 'deinstitutionalisation'. As an alternative to mental hospitals, many schemes have been improvised and adopted to form the basis of 'community care'. It is evident that relatively few scientific evaluative studies have been conducted on these, and it remains unknown whether, in their essential aspects, these alternative innovations are superior to mental hospitals and whether they can bear the whole burden of patient care that mental hospitals have carried – especially that of the patients with severe and chronic mental disorders.

The present situation in member states shows marked variety, in part attributable to the markedly different stages of transition which are detectable, even within each country, and also to the strongly emotive tone of many reports and discussions of the subject in a number of countries.

From these discussions emerged agreement to proceed to the second stage of the study under COMAC-HSR, which is to prepare a multinational, collaborative research project, based on field studies, from which a broad view can be taken of the extent to which the use of mental hospitals has been reduced and replaced by alternative services. The data obtained by each collaborating centre should be epidemiologically sound, as they will be based on all designated mental health services within a defined geographical area which serve a defined population. The aim of the project will be to assess the need for care and to measure the effect of services provided on the outcome, in terms of clinical state, social functioning, and effect on the family of carers.

Acknowledgements

The Workshop Planning Committee wishes to express its thanks to the members of the Concerted Action Committee on Health Services Research (COMAC-HSR) and to the members of the Planning Group on Mental Health Care; to Dr A. E. Baert of the Commission of the European Communities for his valuable assistance; to the authors, discussants, and participants, who readily gave their time and interest to the preparation and conduct of the workshop; and to Mrs K. Perkins for administrative and secretarial assistance.

Publication of this book was made possible by a generous grant from the Commission of the European Communities.

1 Methodology of evaluative studies in the mental health field

HEINZ HÄFNER and
WOLFRAM AN DER HEIDEN

The main objective of evaluative research in the health field is analysis of the effectiveness of medical, social, and health-policy measures and systems as well as of their costs.

Two levels of evaluation: systems and isolable components

The two main levels at which mental health services research, as a domain of evaluative research, is conducted are, firstly, the evaluation of the mental health sector within a national, regional, or community health service; and, secondly, the evaluation of individual mental health facilities or types of care. The first level is characterised by a system aspect, which means that mental health care is perceived as a component, functioning within a more comprehensive care system. However, the system aspect is usually not considered when the effectiveness of individual services or interventions is investigated. The intervention studied is then separated from its associations with other forms of care: this is the case in clinical trials, for example. Both levels have methodological implications.

The evaluation of national health systems

The more complex a care system, the more complex its qualitative, economic, and particularly its functional goals. Because of this complexity, the evaluation of a particular integral component, e.g. the mental health sector, is the more difficult the more its functions are connected, consecutively or simultaneously, with those of adjacent sectors. An example of consecutive connectedness is the after-care provided by rehabilitative and social services for the socially disabled mentally ill, after discharge from hospital. An example of simultaneous connectedness is the need for both general medical and psychiatric care in cases of attempted suicide by severe intoxication (Fig. 1.1).

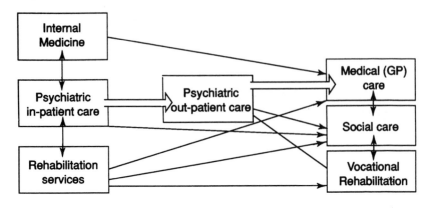

Fig. 1.1. Combination of services and interventions (simplified model)

TABLE 1.1
Mental health care information systems

System of data collection	Missed information about
Continued registration	
Hospital statistics: population based	Multiple contacts
	Complementary services
	Psychiatric out-patient care
	General practice
	Unmet needs (population morbidity)
Case register: population based, case related	Complementary services
	Psychiatric out-patient services
	General practice
	Unmet needs (population morbidity)
Discontinued registration	
General-practice studies	Part of population not in contact
Population studies (including cases in residential care)	

A comprehensive description of the care provided relies upon systems of health data (Table 1.1), which are not limited to subsectors, as hospital statistics are. The structural quality of services can be assessed to a certain extent on the basis of structural indices or conventional norms, such as number of doctors per hospital admission, or beds per unit of accommodation. More difficult is the assessment of aspects of effectiveness, e.g. whether or not the needs of the population served are being met. Waiting lists can be an indication of inadequate organisation or of the insufficient supply of a certain type of care that is needed. Needs for care that are not assessable from utilisation data can only be elucidated, although in a sporadic way, by collecting additional data, e.g. in general-practice or population studies (Wing, 1972).

Evaluation of the functioning of complex systems such as national health services is usually based on rough indicators, e.g. general morbidity and mortality trends, perinatal mortality, the number of avoidable deaths (Holland, 1988), or degree of consumer satisfaction. But it is difficult to find out whether such rough indicators actually reflect the effectiveness of, or deficits in, a health system, or whether they are influenced by other factors such as economic cycles or the health-related behaviour of the population.

The problems posed by a comprehensive evaluation of health services and their mental health components have not yet been solved satisfactorily. Efforts to improve the methods of objective evaluation of the functioning of health systems are urgently required, in view of the high costs of national health systems – although the latter are easier to estimate than the quality of the care supplied.

Monitoring and evaluation of community mental health services

Descriptive analyses of small-scale systems of care, e.g. at the community level, representing national health systems in miniature, provide valuable information for the interpretation of national health care statistics (Wing & Bransby, 1970). At the community level, more detailed, more comprehensive, and case-related data on use of services can be obtained, thus providing a better basis for the understanding of functional associations. Mental health data collected at the community level have substantially contributed to the understanding of changes in the functions of mental health and social services in general, and in the care of the socially disabled mentally ill in particular, during the transition to community-based care (Wing & Hailey, 1972; Wing & Fryers, 1976; Gibbons *et al*, 1984; Häfner, 1985; Häfner & Klug, 1980, 1982; ten Horn *et al*, 1986). In contrast, the functional links between mental-health and other services, although of growing importance in view of the increasing numbers of mentally ill elderly people, have not yet been accorded enough attention.

Continued documentation and analysis of the utilisation of a defined health care system (monitoring) also facilitate its objective control and management. In evaluating the effectiveness and quality of national health services, we find that the only way of supplementing indicator-based models, which are as yet of low reliability, is the description and independent evaluation of components of these systems. An example is the auditing procedure that is used for the evaluation of medical services and their quality by independent experts.

Assessment of the effectiveness of services and interventions

Although the importance cannot be denied of descriptive analysis as a social process of judging the worth of some activity that is free from the pressure of providing evidence of causality (Suchman, 1967), it cannot replace a causal analysis of effectiveness. The latter is particularly indispensable for the assessment of new forms of care, and hence for changing the mental health care system (McInnis & Kitson, 1977). The analysis of a causal relationship between an intervention and an assumed outcome requires consideration of intervening variables, together with the exclusion of possible competing explanations. A prerequisite is the isolation of a clear-cut system, including intervention- and outcome-variables, as well as the use of a design which enables the relevant intervening variables to be controlled for.

These preconditions are usually easier to fulfil when individual services or therapy programmes are being evaluated, but in the evaluation of entire health care programmes, such an approach is generally used without taking account of care delivered by other services or facilities, as a factor that might also account for the effect. This problem can, to a certain extent, be solved by taking a cohort of patients as a starting-point for the investigation, instead of limiting the information about the intervention to a particular programme or service (Fig. 1.2). In this way, all interventions with the patients can be assessed under naturalistic conditions and assigned to individual patients, irrespective of the facility supplying them. This approach is to be recommended especially for the evaluation of the complex care of the socially disabled mentally ill in the community. As Fig. 1.2 shows, in depicting the utilisation behaviour of a cohort of 148 schizophrenic patients over 18 months, such an approach is characterised by marked variations in the frequency and combination of contacts with various services.

Objectives and outcome criteria of mental health care

Evaluating the outcome of an intervention consists of assessing its contribution to the attainment of a defined objective. Central to this approach are the following five characteristics (cf. Weiss, 1972): (a) explicit definition of objectives, (b) defined outcome criteria, (c) measurement of independent, dependent and intervening variables, (d) research design, and (e) evaluation of the whole programme.

Goals

Usually, there is agreement on the general goals of psychiatric care, e.g. 'reduction or containment of mental morbidity' (Wing, 1973). Concrete, operationalised objectives of mental health services are far more difficult to define, but if the global goals of mental health care are not translated into specific operational objectives of a mental health service, it is impossible

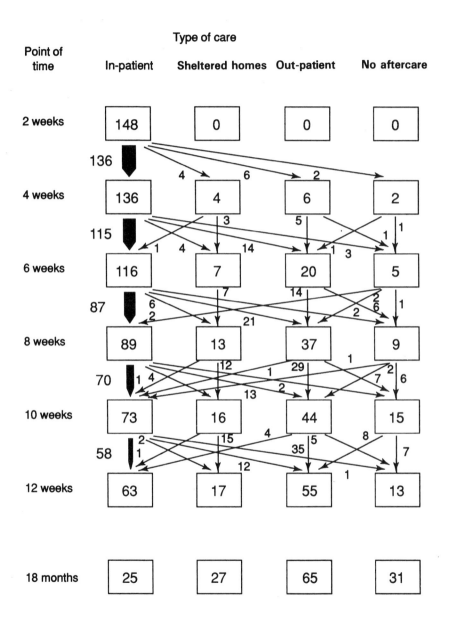

Fig. 1.2. Analysis of patient streams, from Häfner & an der Heiden, (1982)

to define concrete measures for their realisation or assess their effectiveness (Rossi *et al*, 1985). The objectives of many psychiatric services are indeed insufficiently defined (Falloon *et al*, 1987). The reasons are to be looked for, firstly, in the medical tradition, whose standards of defining the objectives of care facilities, e.g. hospitals, have never been high; and, secondly, in the fact that associated with the definition of objectives, especially in mental health care, there is always a statement of social values (Cumming, 1968; Demone *et al*, 1978).

A classic example is the ongoing reform of mental health care. The strongest motive for the reduction or closing of public mental hospitals and the development of complementary services in the community was not the continual protests of psychiatrists, but rather, the inhumane conditions in mental hospitals. This was also the background against which the goals of the reform process, i.e. discharge of long-stay in-patients and provision of alternative extramural care, were defined (Bachrach, 1976). These goals, which continue to guide the policy of several governments, contain implicit value judgements, e.g. that 'life in the community is of higher quality for all mentally ill people than life in a mental hospital'. This is true for all those patients who are capable of leading a better life outside hospital, but we do not yet know exactly what proportion is accounted for by these patients. However, this proportion will be determined not only by the level of disease symptoms of the hospital patients, but also by the living conditions of those who have been discharged into the community.

With the goals described above, the reduction of in-patient activities was laid down as an operative objective of mental health services. As a consequence, indices of in-patient treatment became the most frequently used outcome criterion in mental health services research, and readmission to hospital a synonym for 'relapse' or 'recidivism' (Herz & Melville, 1980; Falloon *et al*, 1983; Falloon, 1984). This development was supported by economic factors: in-patient treatment is, in principle, the most expensive form of care, and reduction of its share in total care is therefore seen as desirable, since it seems, *eo ipso*, to reduce costs.

Output indicators

Indices of in-patient treatment, such as readmissions, are indispensable indicators of the process of care. Their function as output indicators – in the sense of improved mental health or social skills – is, however, to be doubted. Decisions on hospital admission or discharge are not influenced by the mental state of a patient alone. In the case of socially disabled mentally ill persons in particular, they are influenced by the availability of financial and social resources and acceptance on the part of the community population, on the one hand, and hospital factors such as bed capacity and discharge policy, on the other. A better adjustment of treatment objectives to the needs of patients, however, requires the expansion of outcome criteria. Besides the 'care' indices, level of symptoms, degree of social functioning, and consumer satisfaction as an indicator of quality of life are also to be taken into account. In the majority of evaluative studies of mental health services, the three care indices discussed below are used. They are all related to in-patient treatment and are only indirectly, if at all, associated with indices of mental health.

(a) Readmission or readmission rates, from the point of view of the operational objective of aftercare, i.e. reduction of readmissions to in-patient care (cf. Mayer *et al*, 1973; Franklin *et al*, 1975; Kirk, 1976; McCranie & Mizell, 1978; Nuehring *et al*, 1980); point in time and length of readmission are not considered here.

(b) Length of in-patient treatment per time unit (cf. Byers *et al*, 1979; Dincin & Witheridge, 1982). This measure is relevant for its cost aspect, and expresses the length of absence from normal social functioning. As an outcome measure, it is based on the assumption that a successful intervention stabilises the patient's mental state, so that, when re-admission occurs, more rapid restoration to health, and consequently an earlier discharge, becomes possible.

(c) Time spent outside hospital before readmission (cf. Kirk, 1976; Beard *et al*, 1978; Solomon *et al*, 1984). As this criterion is complementary to length of in-patient treatment, a similar association with outcome is assumed, i.e. the intervention under study stabilises the patient's mental state and, in doing so, delays readmission.

These three outcome indices differ in their value in evaluation of the effectiveness of mental health services (Fig. 1.3). In the first place, additional assumptions must be fulfilled. Secondly, the less informative the indices used, the more of their validity is lost by conclusions drawn on the basis of these indices. With the criterion 'number of in-patient readmissions', single readmissions, whose length is not taken into account, can be classified as more favourable than repeated readmissions, but this presupposes that changes in the number of readmissions are not offset by a shortening or prolonging length of stay. Specifically, the classification of single readmissions that prove to be of long duration as good outcomes must be avoided.

When indices (b) and (c) are combined, the problems discussed above become less pronounced. These indices allow a precise operationalisation of the assumed outcome, without requiring additional assumptions about frequency, point in time, and length of readmission. As far as the assumption about the stabilising effect on mental state of the intervention under study is concerned, the use of the two indices, i.e. time spent in the community before readmission and length of stay in hospital after readmission, allows

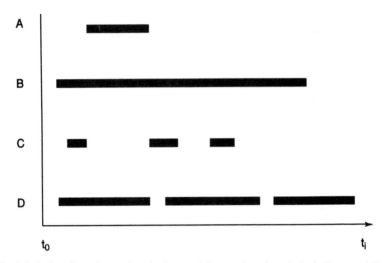

Fig. 1.3. Indices of in-patient care in evaluative research (▬▬ = in-patient episode, A–D = types of disease course). Characteristic feature: (a) Number or rate of readmissions to in-patient care: A and B are regarded as more favourable than C and D; length of stay is not considered. (b) Total length of in-patient episodes: A and C are regarded as more favourable than B and D; number of readmissions is not considered. (c) Length of stay in the community before readmission: in combination with no. 2, sufficient assessment of disease course possible.

the necessary distinction between the two spheres of effect to be made. The latter index, i.e. length of in-patient treatment, is presumably determined by other disease variables, as well as by hospital variables, rather than by length of stay in the community, as our own study showed (Fig. 1.4; Häfner & an der Heiden, 1989a). The additional measure of the outcome criterion, 'total length of in-patient treatment', alone does not pay attention to the point in time of readmission, nor does it distinguish between frequent readmission ('revolving door') and extended stay in hospital. Our own results, drawn from a representative cohort of schizophrenic patients placed in the community, revealed a significant effect of complementary care on the interval prior to the first admission, but no effect at all on length of stay after readmission (Häfner & an der Heiden, 1989a).

Design

Comparative studies of different forms of mental health care are faced with the difficulty of compensating for the lack of knowledge about, or the absence of opportunities of, evaluating individual therapies, within the framework of a mental health care programme. This is usually done by making assumptions about the homogeneity of the care delivered. Both an out-patient

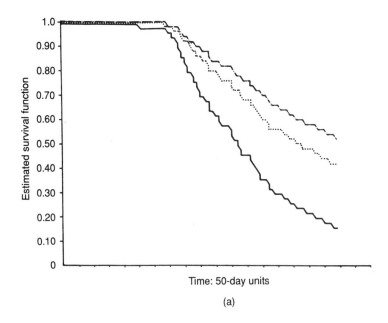

(a)

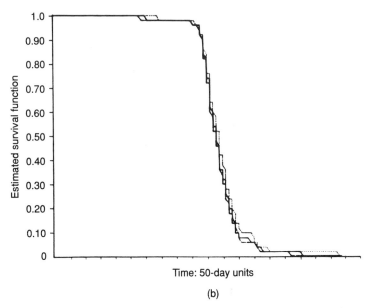

(b)

Fig. 1.4. Length of stay (estimated survival function) in (a) the community and (b) hospital, and share of out-patient medical care (- · - · high, · · · · · medium, ——— low), from Häfner & an der Heiden (1989a)

contact and an in-patient episode must be subsumed under a category of care, irrespective of the treatment or therapy actually administered. In order to be able at least to draw sufficiently plausible conclusions about the outcome of complex programmes of care, we must study groups of patients characterised by more or less homogeneous needs. It is hardly possible to interpret differences in the outcomes of the care provided for heterogenous groups, such as patients discharged from hospital with manifold diagnoses, although such data still predominate in the evaluation of mental health services.

For the mental health services studied, the appropriateness of the care provided is of special importance. In evaluative studies, it is often not possible to guarantee that every patient receives the care that would meet his or her specific needs. Wing *et al*, for example, showed as early as 1972 that forms of occupational therapy can make excessive demands upon a chronically ill person, and thus have an unfavourable effect.

Consequently, the prerequisites for a useful evaluation of any type of care are as follows:

(a) The use of a standardised treatment programme, whose specific active components are defined. If this is impossible, as in the case of studies of 'natural' systems of care, the treatment programme must at least be clearly described, with all its active components.

(b) The active components of the programme must be administered appropriately, i.e., only when indicated.

(c) There must be a guarantee that differences in outcome are not accounted for by other factors; e.g., good hospital care is usually better than low-standard complementary care (Häfner & an der Heiden, 1989*b*), so that the two would not be comparable.

The factors influencing outcome can be distinguished by their contents, type of effects, time of occurrence, and persistence of the changes they produced. The acute effect of pharmacotherapy can be expected to occur within a few days or weeks, whereas occupational training frequently becomes effective only after months. These facts have implications not only for the length of the administration of an intervention, but also for the time-point of the measurement of outcome.

The core question of an evaluation design, i.e. the assessment of effects, must be described in detail, and the method selected must be well founded (Rossi, 1982). Of particular importance are the control, and hence exclusion, of rival explanations. A study is said to possess internal validity if it is possible to explain changes observed in one variable by changes in another variable. A prerequisite is that the factors capable of producing measurable changes in the dependent variable are controlled for. External validity refers to the applicability of the results obtained to conditions outside the study setting.

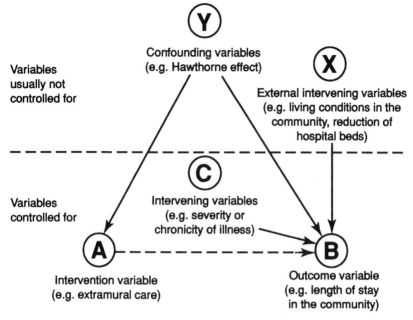

Fig. 1.5. Model of a design for the evaluation of causal effects, from Häfner & an der Heiden (1989b)

To achieve this aim requires populations, variables, and situational conditions that are representative.

The aim of the evaluation of extramural programmes is to elucidate the influence of treatment facilities or interventions on the course of disease. In this context, four categories of factors influencing outcome can be distinguished (Häfner & an der Heiden, 1989*b*) (Fig. 1.5):

(a) Firstly, the intervention under study (in our model, the independent variable denoted by *A*), whose influence on the dependent variable *B* is being investigated.

(b) The second category includes variables (*C*) that do not correlate with the independent variable, but exert an influence on the dependent variable *B*, 'Need for in-patient care'. A group of variables of this category – denoted by *X* in our model – are left unconsidered in the majority of evaluative studies. An example is the reduction of hospital beds, practised purely administratively in many places and resulting in a shortened average length of stay, irrespective of therapeutic success.

(c) The third category contains confounding variables (*Y*) that correlate with both the dependent variable and the independent variable, 'Extramural care'. A typical example is the 'Hawthorne effect' of model programmes, which leads to effects that are not reproducible under normal conditions.

Variables of category (b) determine internal validity, whereas variables of category (c) influence external validity, and hence, the generalisation of the results. A central objective of evaluative studies should be the control of all relevant variables, if possible.

The (quasi-)experimental approach

The classic design for the elimination of the influence of intervening variables in causal analysis of outcome is the experiment. Newcombe (1988) therefore recommends that the classic 'randomised clinical trial' should be adopted as a norm in all evaluative studies of mental health care. But this is wishful thinking.

The simplest type of experiment is to set up various conditions of care, and to measure their effects on outcome variables. At least one of these conditions, in the form of no-treatment controls, serves to enhance the validity of the results concerning the actual treatment effects. In order to eliminate further confounding factors, randomisation is used. The aim of the random allocation of patients between the experimental and control groups is to obtain a study population that is homogeneous in respect of all additionally relevant characteristics at the outset of the investigation. But random allocation of some patients to presumably inferior treatment programmes or to placebo treatment in particular, is increasingly being criticised for ethical reasons.

The naturalistic approach

Not least because of the problems discussed above, observational studies based on a naturalistic design play an important role in the evaluation of mental health services. Keenan (1975) argues with reason that non-experimental research strategies can well come up to scientific standards, frequently being the only possible and effective approach to studying the issues in question. The following three approaches can be applied.

In the first approach, the patients under study are grouped *a posteriori* into two or more subgroups, according to the occurrence or frequency of an event relevant to the assessment of treatment outcome, e.g. readmission to in-patient treatment; these subgroups are then studied for significant differences in their previous use of services. For example, Nuehring *et al* (1980) studied patients with and without readmissions to in-patient treatment over an observation period of six months, with respect to the continuity of previous out-patient treatment (no contacts/'drop-out'/continued treatment; cf. also Christensen, 1974; Franklin *et al*, 1975).

The second approach consists of the observation of a group of patients with respect to their utilisation of selected services over a certain period of time. Depending on the data obtained, the total group is divided into two or more subgroups, which are then compared in terms of outcome criteria. Anthony & Buell (1973), for example, studied the effectiveness of extramural care after in-patient treatment, by comparing a group of patients who had had at least one contact with an aftercare clinic with another group who had been without aftercare. McCranie & Mizell (1978) compared the readmission rates of three groups of patients who differed in their frequency of contacts with an aftercare clinic (cf. also Kirk, 1976; Solomon *et al*, 1984).

Finally, there is a group of studies directly comparing the effects of the utilisation of different services with one another (e.g. Vitale & Steinbach, 1965). It is to this group that, for example, the attempt to evaluate the run-down of two large-scale mental hospitals in London – Friern and Claybury – and the parallel setting up of community-based services belongs (Knapp *et al*, 1990). To achieve this aim, two matched groups from the total group of long-stay patients (length of stay of one year and more) are being compared with one another, i.e. patients discharged to complementary services (group homes, hostels, private landlords, foster homes) on the one hand, and patients remaining in hospital on the other. The comparison of the two groups is expected to provide answers to questions as to whether the clinical status and social competence of the patients undergo changes after discharge, whether their quality of life is improved, and which type of care is less expensive.

The three designs discussed differ in terms of the following three dimensions:

(a) the degree to which situational conditions are controlled for;
(b) the degree of controlling for or randomness in the administration of an intervention;
(c) the inclusion of a control group, representing a random selection from a treatment population, parallelised according to mean values or matched pairwise.

In evaluative studies using a naturalistic design, the problem of controlling for situational conditions and intervening variables is particularly pro-nounced. In such studies, the possibility cannot be ruled out that at the outset of the intervention being studied, the patients already differ in characteristics which, directly or indirectly, influence outcome criteria, and thus limit the generalisation of the results. Zohar *et al* (1987), for example, found that decisions about admissions to in-patient treatment in a hospital located near the community depended not only on disease-related variables, but also on a combination of demographic, clinical, and temporal factors.

The frequent lack of controlling for all factors effective within the scope of studies based on the observation of the 'natural' utilisation of mental health services may be one of the reasons why such studies have so far failed to produce results which would allow consistent conclusions to be drawn about the effectiveness of extramural care in the treatment of chronically mentally ill patients.

Evaluative studies based on a naturalistic design should also aim at the exclusion of possible alternative interpretations. The fact that intervening and confounding variables are not controlled for by random assignment must be counterbalanced by their explicit measurement and the inclusion of assumptions about their effects in the study design. This means that all relevant variables must be carefully assessed, and their contribution to the outcome of an intervention partialled out by using suitable techniques (Häfner & an der Heiden, 1989*c*). The advantage of such a design is its applicability to the natural conditions of complex mental health care programmes, as far as the latter can be sufficiently isolated from more complex systems.

Comparison of mental health care programmes by separate assessment of effectiveness and direct costs

Jones *et al* (1980) followed up two cohorts of first-admitted schizophrenic patients ($n = 55/51$) in Manchester, retrospectively over four years. They compared the global therapies practised in a psychiatric unit of a district general hospital and in an area mental hospital in terms of costs, and clinical and social outcomes. From the results of this study, it can be concluded that a large number of social and illness variables have to be considered, in order to be able to interpret the differences in outcome and costs correctly. However, by comparing the costs and effectiveness of different therapeutic strategies administered to the same target populations, we should be able to determine which programme involves the lower costs.

Direct costs as an indicator of appropriate care

By studying representative populations of chronic schizophrenics, Hess *et al* (1986) in Berne (Switzerland) and Häfner *et al* (1986) in Mannheim (Germany) compared the costs of the total network of extramural services offered in defined catchment areas with those of continued psychiatric hospital care, on the basis of directly measurable costs of medical, psychiatric, and social services. Both studies showed that the costs of extramural care, including readmission when relapses occurred, were more than 50% lower than the costs of continued hospital care (Fig. 1.6).

However, by analysing the distribution of the costs per case, Häfner *et al* showed that the findings are applicable only under certain conditions. With increasing proportions of chronically ill and disabled patients in extramural care, the costs of extramural care per case, and consequently the average costs, increase. This is because the more intensive care of the

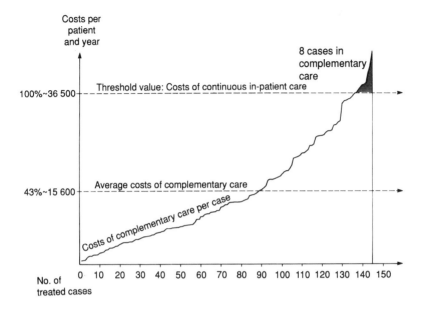

Fig. 1.6. Direct costs of community care (based on prices in 1980), from Häfner et al (1986)

severely ill and disabled, recently discharged, produces considerably higher costs than does that of less severely disabled patients who are discharged from hospital before them. At the same time, the psychiatric in-patient population changes, as fewer slightly ill but increasing numbers of severely ill patients, producing higher costs, are admitted.

Obviously, this system aspect of mental health services is an important frame of reference for the generalisation of results of small-scale evaluative studies, which may select different sectors of the continuum of severity of illness or disablement for the care programme that is being measured. In order to apply the results of such studies to the target group of all the socially disabled of a particular category, we must take into account the system aspect, by employing an epidemiological design. This can be accomplished by, for example, comparing the study population and the total target group served in the same catchment area in terms of relevant variables, by using simultaneously collected case register data. A comprehensive and continuous documentation of the utilisation of the whole network of services by the population of a catchment area thus becomes of decisive importance, if results yielded by studies covering only selected patient groups and limited time periods are to be interpreted.

Conclusions

Although the problems posed by the evaluation of mental health services are greater, the more complex the programmes or systems investigated, there are enough appropriate methods and research designs available to extend promising paths into the thicket of unanswered questions. The investigation of the effectiveness of small-scale, less complex systems makes a contribution not only to the mosaic of knowledge, but also to an understanding of the functioning and effectiveness of the complex systems which they reflect in a simplified form.

References

ANTHONY, W. A. & BUELL, G. J. (1973) Psychiatric aftercare effectiveness as a function of patient demographic characteristics. *Journal of Consulting and Clinical Psychology*, **41**, 116–119.

BACHRACH, L. L. (1976) A note on some recent studies of released mental hospital patients in the community. *American Journal of Psychiatry*, **133**, 73–75.

BEARD, J. H., MALAMUD, T. J. & ROSSMAN, E. (1978) Psychiatric rehabilitation and long-term rehospitalization rates: the findings of two research studies. *Schizophrenia Bulletin*, **4**, 622–635.

BYERS, E. S., COHEN, S. H. & HARSHBARGER, D. D. (1979) The quantity and quality of aftercare services: relationship with recidivism in mental health patients. *Canadian Journal of Behavioral Sciences*, **11**, 11–20.

CHRISTENSEN, K. J. (1974) A 5-year follow-up study of male schizophrenics: evaluation of factors influencing success and failure in the community. *Acta Psychiatrica Scandinavica*, **50**, 60–72.

CUMMING, J. H. (1968) Some criteria for evaluation. In *Comprehensive Mental Health: The Challenge of Evaluation*, (eds L.M. Roberts, N. Greenfield & M. Miller), pp. 29–40. Madison, WI: University of Wisconsin Press.

DEMONE, H. W., SCHULBERG, H. C. & BROSKOWSKI, A. (1978) Evaluation in the context of developments in human services. In *Evaluation of Human Service Programs*, (eds C. C. Attkisson, W. A. Hargreaves, M. J. Horowitz, *et al*), pp. 27–41. New York: Academic Press.

DINCIN, J. & WITHERIDGE, T. F. (1982) Psychiatric rehabilitation as a deterrent to recidivism. *Hospital and Community Psychiatry*, **33**, 645–650.

FALLOON, I., WILKINSON, G., BURGESS, J., *et al* (1987) Evaluation in psychiatry: planning, developing, and evaluating community-based mental health services for adults. In *Evaluating Mental Health Practice: Methods and Applications*, (ed. D. Milne), pp. 203–238. London: Croom Helm.

FALLOON, I. R. H. (1984) Relapse: a reappraisal of assessment of outcome in schizophrenia. *Schizophrenia Bulletin*, **10**, 293–299.

———, MARSHAL, G. N., BOYD, J. L., *et al* (1983) Relapse in schizophrenia: a review of the concept and its definitions. *Psychological Medicine*, **13**, 469–477.

FRANKLIN, J. L., KITTREDGE, L. D. & THRASHER, J. H. (1975) A survey of factors related to mental hospital readmissions. *Hospital and Community Psychiatry*, **26**, 749–751.

GIBBONS, J., JENNINGS, C. & WING, J. K. (1984) *Psychiatric Care in Eight Register Areas, 1976–1981*. Psychiatric Case Register, Fareham: Knowle Hospital.

HÄFNER, H. (1985) Changing patterns of mental health care. *Acta Psychiatrica Scandinavica*, **71** (suppl. 319), 151–164.

——— & AN DER HEIDEN, W. (1982) Evaluation gemeindenaher Versorgung psychisch Kranker. *Archiv für Psychiatrie und Nervenkrankheiten*, **232**, 71–95.

——— & ——— (1989a) The evaluation of mental health care systems. *British Journal of Psychiatry*, **155**, 12–17.

—— & —— (1989*b*) Evaluation of care for the disabled mentally ill: theoretical issues. *European Archives of Psychiatry and Neurological Sciences*, **238**, 179–184.

—— & —— (1989*c*) Effectiveness and cost of community care for schizophrenic patients. *Hospital and Community Psychiatry*, **40**, 59–63.

——, ——, BUCHHOLZ, W., *et al* (1986) Organisation, Wirksamkeit und Wirtschaftlichkeit komplementärer Versorgung Schizophrener. *Nervenarzt*, **57**, 214–226.

—— & KLUG, J. (1980) Der Aufbau einer gemeindenahen Versorgung in Mannheim – erste Ergebnisse einer wissenschaftlichen Begleitung. In *Psychiatrie 5 Jahre nach der Enquete*, (eds H. Häfner & W. Picard), Aktion Psychisch Kranke e.V. Tagungsberichte, vol. 5, pp. 29–42. Köhn: Rheinland Verlag.

—— & —— (1982) The impact of an expanding community mental health service on patterns of bed usage: evaluation of a four-year period of implementation. *Psychological Medicine*, **12**, 177–190.

HERZ, M. I. & MELVILLE, C. (1980) Relapse in schizophrenia. *American Journal of Psychiatry*, **137**, 801–805.

HESS, D., CIOMPI, L. & DAUWALDER, H. (1986) Nutzen- und Kosten-Evaluation eines sozialpsychiatrischen Dienstes. *Nervenarzt*, **57**, 204–213.

HOLLAND, W. W. (ed.) (1988) *European Communities Atlas of Avoidable Death*. Commission of the European Communities Health Services Research Series no. 3. Oxford: Oxford University Press.

JONES, R., GOLDBERG, D. & HUGHES, B. (1980) A comparison of two different services treating schizophrenia: a cost-benefit approach. *Psychological Medicine*, **10**, 493–505.

KEENAN, B. (1975) Designing mental health studies: the pragmatics of nonexperimental design. *Hospital and Community Psychiatry*, **26**, 739–740.

KIRK, S. A. (1976) Effectiveness of community services for discharged mental hospital patients. *American Journal of Orthopsychiatry*, **46**, 646–659.

KNAPP, M., BEECHAM, J., ANDERSON, J. G., *et al* (1990) The TAPS project. 3: predicting the community costs of closing psychiatric hospitals. *British Journal of Psychiatry*, **157**, 661–670.

MAYER, J. E., HOTZ, M. & ROSENBLATT, A. (1973) The readmission patterns of patients referred to aftercare clinics. *Journal of the Bronx State Hospital*, **1**, 180–188.

McCRANIE, E. W. & MIZELL, T. A. (1978) Aftercare for psychiatric patients: does it prevent rehospitalization? *Hospital and Community Psychiatry*, **29**, 584–587.

McINNIS, T. & KITSON, L. (1977) Process evaluation in mental health systems. *International Journal of Mental Health*, **5**, 58–72.

NEWCOMBE, R. G. (1988) Evaluation of treatment effectiveness in psychiatric research. *British Journal of Psychiatry*, **152**, 696–697.

NUEHRING, E. M., THAYER, J. H. & LADNER, R. A. (1980) On the factors predicting rehospitalization among two state mental hospital patient populations. *Administration in Mental Heath*, **7**, 247–270.

ROSSI, P. H. (1982) *Standards for Evaluation Practice*. San Francisco, CA: Jossey-Bass.

——, FREEMAN, H. E. & WRIGHT, S. R. (1985) *Evaluation: A Systematic Approach*. Beverly Hills, CA: Sage.

SOLOMON, P., DAVIS, J. & GORDON, B. (1984) Discharged state hospital patients' characteristics and use of aftercare: effect on community tenure. *American Journal of Psychiatry*, **141**, 1566–1570.

SUCHMAN, E. A. (1967) *Evaluative Research: Principles and Practice in Public Health Service and Social Action Programs*. New York: Russell Sage Foundation.

TEN HORN, G. H. M. M., GIEL, R., GULBINAT, W. H., *et al* (1986) *Psychiatric Case Registers in Public Health*. Amsterdam: Elsevier.

VITALE, J. H. & STEINBACH, M. (1965) The prevention of relapse of chronic mental patients. *International Journal of Social Psychiatry*, **11**, 85–95.

WEISS, C. H. (1972) *Evaluation Research*. Englewood Cliffs, NJ: Prentice-Hall.

WING, J. K. (1972) Principles of evaluation. In *Evaluating a Community Psychiatric Service: The Camberwell Register, 1964–1971*, (eds J. K. Wing & A. M. Hailey), pp. 11–39. London: Oxford University Press.

18   *Wing*

—— (1973) Principles of evaluation. In *Roots of Evaluation*, (eds J. K. Wing & A. M. Hailey), pp. 3–12. London: Oxford University Press.

—— & BRANSBY, R. (eds) (1970) Psychiatric case registers. DHSS Statistical Report Series no. 8. London: HMSO.

—— & FRYERS, T. (1976) Psychiatric services in Camberwell and Salford. Statistics from the Camberwell and Salford psychiatric registers, 1964–1974. MRC Social Psychiatry Unit, London, and Department of Community Medicine, Manchester.

—— & HAILEY, A. M. (eds) (1972) *Evaluating a Community Psychiatric Service: The Camberwell Register, 1964–1971*. London: Oxford University Press.

WING, L., WING, J. K., STEVENS, B., *et al* (1972) An epidemiological and experimental evaluation of industrial rehabilitation of chronic patients in the community. In *Evaluating a Community Psychiatric Service: The Camberwell Register, 1964–1971*, (eds J. K. Wing & A. M. Hailey), pp. 283–308. London: Oxford University Press.

ZOHAR, M., HADAZ, Z. & MODAN, B. (1987) Factors affecting the decision to admit mental patients in a community hospital. *Journal of Nervous and Mental Disease*, **175**, 301–305.

Discussion: JOHN K. WING

The broad context of health care

This excellent presentation begins with a proper injunction to consider mental health services as only one part of a larger system of health care. We should remember that the basic philosophy of the originators of the social welfare systems that are characteristic of many countries in Europe was that prevention is better than cure. Underpinning the services specifically devoted to illness, there are many forms of social support and care that are intended to promote the welfare of all citizens, whether ill or not.

Though the philosophy of prevention through social welfare measures has obvious practical limitations, two end-point examples may serve to illustrate its relevance to our topic. No description of residential facilities for the mentally ill is complete without some attempt to take account of the availability of low-cost accommodation of reasonable quality to people (particularly those who are poor and unmarried) who are *not* mentally ill. Similarly, the provision of a wide range of employment opportunities to suit all levels of ability should provide a foundation on which to build more specific services for those who are disabled in various ways.

This background network of social support services cannot be complete, though some countries manage better than others. An index of deprivation is a useful means of identifying geographical areas of particular concern. Figure 1.1 is taken from a recent publication from eight UK Psychiatric Case Registers (Wing, J. K., 1989*a*). It shows the population growth or decline in the districts covered during the 60 years from 1921 to 1981. Oxford, for example, doubled its population in this period, while that of Camberwell was halved. I have added the Jarman index of deprivation for the Health Districts concerned (Jarman, 1983, 1984; Hirsch, 1988).

Dual hypotheses may be put forward that attractive areas acquire relatively healthy newcomers, while deprived areas not only suffer from out-migration, but may also have an attraction for people with mental health problems. There is a danger of oversimplification if the many other factors involved in producing these complex statistical indices are not also considered, a task which cannot be done here. But it has long been a truism of psychiatric epidemiology that indices of social isolation are particularly useful in identifying vulnerable areas.

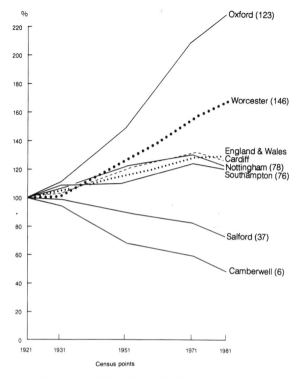

Fig. 1.7. *Percentage population change (1921–81) in health districts with contrasting Jarman indices of deprivation (lower Jarman index = greater deprivation)*

The relevance of such facts for planners might appear to be obvious, but they have not always been taken into account when generalising from the results of evaluating services in one area to recommendations for planning elsewhere.

Top-down and bottom-up approaches to evaluation

However, most of what Häfner & an der Heiden say here is concerned with more direct methods of assessment of mental health services. We can approach the problems involved from two very different perspectives – top-down and bottom-up. The first perspective is administrative, or 'monitoring', in which the indices used imply value, but do not test it. The information needed is relatively 'hard' and simple to acquire routinely, but it has only a statistical relationship to individual need. It can even be misleading.

The other perspective is personal and can be directed much more closely at an evaluation of whether needs are really being met in individual cases, but this is time-consuming and costly, and the information gathered tends to be soft, complex, full of value judgements, and difficult to generalise from. The two conceptual time scales are also different. It is therefore rational for planners to prefer the top-down approach, which is quick and convenient, and which leaves interpretation (including value judgements) to them. Clinicians and consumers, also rationally, tend to prefer the bottom-up mode.

B

A key question about the possibility of the practical evaluation of services that exercises me is whether the two perspectives can be combined – whether a bottom-up needs-assessment system can form part of a routine top-down health information system. Before trying to answer this question, I should first underline the distinction, mentioned by the authors, that I have previously drawn between 'care', care 'agents', and service 'settings'. This is basic to clarity of thought about evaluation, even if it is not always easy or possible to achieve. 'Care' includes all forms of personal interventions, from pharmacotherapy through counselling to welfare support. 'Agents' are the people, professional and informal, who provide the care. 'Settings' comprise the various structures in which the care is given. The three terms should be understood as being in quotation marks, in order to emphasise their differential significance.

Aims, and designs for assessing whether aims are achieved

Evaluation must begin with a statement of the aims that are intended to be achieved. From the research worker's point of view, they can be seen as hypotheses, to be tested against other possible assumptions. Planners, clinicians, and consumers may all have different, even conflicting aims. I was particularly pleased to note that Häfner & an der Heiden used the concept of social disablement, rather than diagnosis, as the central concept in evaluation. I suspect we should all be on common ground if our most fundamental aim was stated to be to prevent or minimise the social disablement associated with mental illness by dealing with its major components – disease, disability, disadvantage, and distress or demoralisation. Each factor can be measured but, like Häfner & an der Heiden, I shall not try to cover that immense topic here (Wing, J. K., 1989*b*, 1990). I would, however, add a rider to the overall aim, to the effect that the more severe the social disablement, the higher the priority that needs should be met.

The concept of 'quality of life', is mentioned in this paper only in the context of consumer satisfaction. One must be very careful in using that as an index of quality, unless the consumer is fully aware of the richness and variety of the range of residential, occupational, and recreational options that ought to be available. If impairments prevent an individual from making use of other, unimpaired, talents, 'enabling' interventions are required in order that these potentials can be realised. This may include, within the network of 'settings' that form a comprehensive community psychiatric service, the provision of sheltered environments of various kinds to enhance the quality of life.

Fortunately, pioneer consumer associations such as the National Schizophrenia Fellowship and the National Autistic Society have provided a lead that has been followed by organisations across the whole of Europe. Evaluators can learn a great deal from them about the quality of life of persons afflicted by severe and persistent mental illness and also that of their families.

When the aims are translated into terms of preventing admission to hospital, or increasing the number of day-care places, or providing sheltered, low-cost apartments, the intentions are clear enough, but it cannot be assumed that fulfilling these targets will, *ipso facto*, reduce social disablement or improve quality of life. Some evidence to that effect has to be forthcoming.

Sometimes, the value implicit in an index is so obvious and incontrovertible that it would be ridiculous to waste time and energy on sophisticated designs: shortening waiting lists is a case in point. And the wider and more comprehensive the range of choices, given proper organisation and management, the more likely needs are to be, at the least, considered. There is also undoubtedly a case to be made under certain circumstances for highly focused descriptive studies, aimed by independent and well-informed investigators at discovering whether the claims made by a particular group of 'agents' for the effects of 'care' in a particular kind of 'setting' are justified. Nevertheless, monitoring must usually be supplemented by evaluation. Häfner & an der Heiden have described experimental and quasi-experimental design, as well as three types of naturalistic design. Controlled designs are most useful for testing the efficacy of methods of 'care', particularly towards the treatment end of the 'care' spectrum. Leff's trials of family intervention come into this category, as do the trials of home versus hospital care for people with schizophrenia. I agree that it is optimistic to suppose that controlled experiments of service settings will become common, though a few have been carried out (Wing, J. K., 1960; Wing, L., *et al*, 1972; Paykel *et al*, 1982; Hyde *et al*, 1987).

Naturalistic designs, as Häfner & an der Heiden argue, do not have to lack rigour. On the contrary, they depend on the wit of the research worker to incorporate as many independent checks as can be conceived and, above all, on a comparison between properly selected samples. There are plenty of good examples, the main problem being that replication is hard to perform.

I would particularly commend a study that started in the MRC Social Psychiatry Unit in 1980 and still has a year or more to run in the successor unit. It is concerned with the run-down to closure of a hospital for the mentally retarded. The matched-control succeeded by self-control design mentioned by Häfner & an der Heiden was adopted. During the first five years of the project, residents were moved out of hospital to whatever apparently suitable alternative accommodation could be found. During the second phase, which ended with the closure of the hospital in August 1988, new, purpose-built accommodation was provided. The results of research on the first phase have now been published (Wing, L., 1989), and they make compelling reading for anyone who is interested in objective analysis and comment. Because the problems of sampling are somewhat less complicated than those posed by long-term mental illness, a map of the issues posed in undertaking such crucial tests of current policies is very clearly laid out before the reader.

The concept of 'need'

A central concept in the paper under discussion, which draws upon all the disparate elements of evaluative research, is that of 'need'; it provides the link between problem, action, and evaluation. The most common criticism of the concept is that it fails to distinguish between statements of fact and statements of value. But this itself is the central problem in any application of research results. It is impossible to leave value out.

I first quoted Graham Matthew's clear and economical definitions (1971) of the basic terms 'need', 'demand', and 'utilisation' 19 years ago (Wing, J. K., 1972), and have repeated them many times since:

> "A need for medical care exists when an individual has an illness or disability for which there is effective and acceptable treatment or care. It can be defined either in terms of the type of illness or disability causing the need or of the treatment or facilities for treatment required to meet it. A demand for care exists when an individual considers that he has a need and wishes to receive care. Utilization occurs when an individual actually receives care. Need is not necessarily expressed as demand, and demand is not necessarily followed by utilization, while, on the other hand, there can be demand and utilization without real underlying need for the particular service used."

These definitions were intended for general medical services, but, with a few modifications, they will do very well for the equivalent problems met when assessing psychiatric services. Each can be measured.

Most evaluations using a concept of need have been made in global terms, with one or more clinicians or research workers, in effect, making private judgements as to the kind of care and service thought to be necessary. Detailed measurements of clinical and social characteristics which are likely to allow a degree of repeatability between studies, are often provided, but the paths from these problems to the action regarded as appropriate are not publicly specified (e.g. Leff & Vaughn, 1972; Mann & Cree, 1976; Leach & Wing, 1980; Wykes, 1982; Wykes *et al*, 1982).

A recent pilot study of a more sophisticated needs-assessment system has suggested that it could prove useful for evaluating and comparing services (Brewin *et al*, 1987; Brewin & Wing, 1988). These procedures mimic those of a multidisciplinary team with responsibility for providing a service, without being limited to prescribing only those methods of 'care', professional and informal 'agents', and service 'settings' that are actually available. The methods of assessment and rules of allocation of interventions and facilities diminish subjectivity and increase comparability between studies. Substantially more specification could be attained, particularly on the indications for various forms of treatment. The element of value involved in making decisions about needs is to that extent reduced. Moreover, decision points are publicly specified and criticisable. Systems of this kind require much further development, however. Experience should lead to improvements and adaptations to the needs of people with other types of problem, and it should also be relatively simple to add the costs of items of service.

The next challenge is to adapt this kind of research system, now implemented on a laptop computer, to the practical exigencies of clinical practice, in order that it could be built into a District Health and Social Information System, which would combine the advantages of the top-down and bottom-up perspectives. It would, of course, be necessary to make sure that it did not combine the disadvantages instead. The solution to the problem of practicality, as Rohde has pointed out, is to ensure that the system rewards all those who operate and use it, from administrators to ward staff to clerks to patients. His CRISP system bids fair to meet this basic criterion.

Field studies proposal

Finally, there are the opportunities for cross-European research. It does seem sensible, as the European Medical Research Council has suggested, to make comparisons among the rich variety of patterns of services available, in order to draw conclusions that might enable us to achieve our aims better. I would urge that long-term social disablement associated with mental illness be the principal focus of these. If our communities can provide proper care and a decent standard of living for this group, without inflicting secondary disabilities on them, the rest of the network of services will more readily fall into place.

The design of such a study must be most carefully considered. The chief problem is to identify people who either are, or are at high risk of becoming, socially disabled. Straightforward sampling of candidates for admission to hospital will not guarantee that, nor will the usual diagnostic criteria. At the risk of oversimplification, I would say that it is not until at least ten years into the course of disorders like schizophrenia that the chronicity of disablement becomes sufficiently apparent to be made the basis for sampling. But comparative studies of how these problems are dealt with in different countries should prove highly rewarding, if only the sampling problems can be solved.

References

BREWIN, C. R., WING, J. K., MANGEN, S., *et al* (1987) Principles and practice of measuring needs in the long-term mentally ill: the MRC Needs for Care Assessment. *Psychological Medicine*, **17**, 971–981.

—— & —— (1988) *The MRC Needs for Care Assessment Manual* (2nd edn). MRC Social Psychiatry Unit.

HIRSCH, S. R. (Chairman) (1988) *Psychiatric Beds and Resources: Factors Influencing Bed Use and Service Planning*. London: Gaskell.

HYDE, C., BRIDGES, K., GOLDBERG, D., *et al* (1987) The evaluation of a hostel ward. A controlled study using modified cost-benefit analysis. *British Journal of Psychiatry*, **151**, 805–812.

JARMAN, B. (1983) Identification of underprivileged areas. *British Medical Journal*, **286**, 1705–1709.

—— (1984) Validation and distribution of scores. *British Medical Journal*, **289**, 1587–1592.

LEACH, J. & WING, J. K. (1980) *Helping Destitute Men*. London: Tavistock.

LEFF, J. L. & VAUGHN, C. (1972) Psychiatric patients in-contact and out-of-contact with services: a clinical and social assessment. In *Evaluating a Community Psychiatric Service. The Camberwell Register, 1964–1971*, (eds J. K. Wing & A. M. Hailey), pp. 259–274. London: Oxford University Press.

MANN, S. A. & CREE, W. (1976) 'New' long-stay psychiatric patients. A national sample of 15 hospitals in England and Wales, 1972–3. *Psychological Medicine*, **6**, 603–616.

MATTHEW, G. K. (1971) Measuring need and evaluating services. In *Portfolio for Health. Problems and Progress in Medical Care*, (ed. G. McLachlan), (6th series). London: Oxford University Press.

PAYKEL, E. S., MANGEN, S. P., GRIFFITH, J. H., *et al* (1982) Community psychiatric nursing for neurotic patients: a controlled trial. *British Journal of Psychiatry*, **140**, 531–581.

WING, J. K. (1960) A pilot experiment on the rehabilitation of long-hospitalised male schizophrenic patients. *British Journal of Preventive and Social Medicine*, **14**, 173–180.

—— (1972) Principles of evaluation. In *Evaluating a Community Psychiatric Service. The Camberwell Register, 1964–1971*, (eds J. K. Wing & A. M. Hailey). London: Oxford University Press.

—— (ed.) (1989a) *Health Services Planning and Research*. London: Gaskell.

—— (1989b) The measurement of social disablement. The MRC social behaviour and social role performance schedules. *Social Psychiatry and Epidemiology*, **24**, 173–178.

—— (1990) Meeting the needs of people with psychiatric disorders. *Social Psychiatry* (January 1990), in press.

WING, L. (1989) *Hospital Closure and the Resettlement of Residents*. London: Avebury/Gower.

——, WING, J. K., STEVENS, B., *et al* (1972) An epidemiological and experimental evaluation of industrial rehabilitation of chronic psychotic patients in the community. In *Evaluating a Community Psychiatric Service. The Camberwell Register, 1964–1971*, (eds J. K. Wing & A. M. Hailey), pp. 283–308. London: Oxford University Press.

WYKES, T. (1982) A hostel-ward for 'new' long-stay patients. An evaluative study of a ward in a house. *Psychological Medicine Monograph* (suppl. 2), pp. 5–55. Cambridge: Cambridge University Press.

——, CREER, C. & STURT, E. (1982) A survey of long-term users of the psychiatric services in Camberwell. *Psychological Medicine Monograph* (suppl. 2), pp. 59–97. Cambridge: Cambridge University Press.

2 Effectiveness of treatment strategies for the chronic mentally ill

MARIANNE KASTRUP

When the word 'effectiveness' is used in health services research, it generally refers to the degree of goal attainment, which in the individual case means whether the psychiatric patient has reached a higher degree of health, has to suffer less, reduces his or her contact with the services, etc. A main goal of any psychiatric treatment strategy is to improve the patient's mental health status and social functioning. In addition, all treatment strategies may attain subsidiary goals, such as reducing the burden on families, changing public opinion, or preventing professional burn-out. Compared to the main goals, these subsidiary goals are of a more diversified nature, and their accomplishment more arduous to evaluate. Nevertheless, their importance should not be underestimated in a discussion of treatment strategies.

Seen in the light of the radical changes that have taken place in mental health services, there is a need to analyse what impact such studies have had on the effectiveness of treatment. What have been the consequences for treatment strategies of the chronic mentally ill? What have been the implications for the psychiatric profession? And what are the unresolved issues related to optimum care of the chronic population?

Historical changes

Until a few decades ago, the large European mental hospitals often provided a low standard of living for the resident population (Häfner, 1987). The hospital environment lacked stimulation, and rehabilitation was slow to take place. Public opinion was persuaded that the mentally ill would be better cared for outside psychiatric institutions. In the process of deinstitutionalisation, several factors have played contributory roles: the introduction of psychopharmacology has been significant, but so have political decisions (Rose, 1979). Politically, it was argued that psychiatric patients were in fact debilitated by long-term hospital care, that an institutionalised form of behaviour was thereby produced, and that, as a result, patients became chronically ill. Following this, there has been a change in the delivery of services that has followed different pathways in the various EC countries, but almost everywhere, overall policy has focused on extramural care instead of hospital care, and replaced long-stay institutional care with short-stay admissions and domiciliary help.

The psychiatric institution

In most European countries, the process of deinstitutionalisation has resulted in a rapid decline in the in-patient population of mental hospitals, and analyses of this policy have tended to present the drop in the number of hospital beds as an evidence of success. Recently, however, there has been a growing awareness of the complexity of the system and of the fact that it is no solution simply to empty the hospitals. There is also an increasing recognition that no matter what the quality and availability of community mental health services, admission to a psychiatric hospital cannot be avoided in all cases. Despite the most vigorous efforts to return patients to the community, a small percentage are likely to require in-patient care for shorter or longer periods.

When this is needed, however, certain minimum requirements should be observed for the standard of the institutions. These include, among the most basic, access to privacy, leisure activities, and outdoor facilities. Experience has shown, however, that such requirements are not automatically met, even when a general improvement in conditions has taken place. The rights of psychiatric patients have to be fought for continually, not only within the psychiatric institution, but also in negotiations with the responsible political authorities. As an example, these requirements were modified to a 'good hospital standard' – whatever that implies – when the Mental Health Act was passed in the Danish Parliament.

The mental health professionals

The shift from hospital to community care has had major implications for the psychiatric profession, and strong feelings have been expressed, both for and against it (Burns, 1988). In Europe, there has been a considerable increase in the number of psychiatrists, both in relation to the general population and to the total number of doctors (Freeman *et al*, 1985). This development is to be welcomed by patients, as well as by their relatives, since the presence of qualified mental health professionals facilitates a diversified treatment approach, in contrast to the former custodial care.

But this discussion should not limit itself to the number of psychiatrists, since, with the community mental health movement, we have simultaneously experienced a development towards interdisciplinary teams, in which the psychiatrist is one of several participating professionals. This has been accompanied by an increasing competence and responsibility being given to non-medical groups. However, experience with mental health teams shows the need for continual supervision and education of these teams, if they are to be successful in managing the degree of psychopathology that is presented by many cases.

The question of professional burn-out is another important issue in the discussion of treatment strategies for the chronically ill. Working with chronic psychotic patients in an environment characterised by limited resources and often under the surveillance of a critical public opinion is a strenuous task. The negative impact these factors have on professional satisfaction, and ultimately on the quality of treatment offered, should not be underestimated. Furthermore, with the establishment of new care facilities and the accompanying therapeutic optimism, a drain of personnel occurs away from institutional care to these various community programmes. Often, it is the younger or more active staff members who take up this challenge, leaving the psychiatric institutions with the older, more traditionally minded members.

The community mental health programme

To set up a community care programme that is, in fact, caring and has anything to do with the community has been shown to be a difficult task (Cohen, 1988). To require that the programme should treat the chronic mentally ill effectively makes this task even more difficult. A first important step to be taken is a survey of the population and catchment area to be served. What is the infrastructure and the socio-demographic profile of the area? What is the attitude of the population towards psychiatric illness and towards the available services? What do we know about the psychiatric morbidity of the area, and are there special precautions to be taken in developing the service? Some energy should be directed towards efforts to change public attitudes towards psychiatric illness and encourage acceptance of patients' needs and behaviour in the community. One way may be to offer educational programmes, or to arrange 'open house' meetings. Information about the availability of both social services and voluntary agencies which can be used by people with chronic illnesses should be publicised.

During the next phase, that of implementation, data need to be collected in order to monitor the execution of the programme. This may take place in various stages and is followed by the final phase: evaluation, in which an ongoing assessment is needed of the various stages and of the outcome seen in relation to the objectives of the programme. As pointed out by Häfner & an der Heiden (1989), evaluative studies of the effectiveness of community psychiatric care are often contradictory with respect to outcome. In order to avoid that and to provide reliable results, they emphasise the need to describe the interventions that are subject to evaluation, to study homogeneous patient populations with respect to the relevance of the therapeutic interventions and outcome variables, and to have clear definitions of the therapeutic objectives.

When different kinds of services are compared, outcome is frequently measured in terms of number of readmissions, length of admissions, and time spent outside institutional care. However, in the case of the chronically ill, these measures are in many ways unsatisfactory. To avoid hospital care is not in itself a positive aim to be attempted under all circumstances. In order to evaluate and compare different services, information is needed on the limiting factors and negative consequences such as homelessness, stigmatisation, poor social functioning, low quality of life, and the burden on the families.

As pointed out by Cohen (1988), it is important to acknowledge the diversity of community care. The aim is that with optimal care, the patient will experience a higher quality of life within the community, the family will not feel imposed upon, and the community will also feel that it has gained. In practice, it is not an easy task to deal with such complex factors in evaluating a programme that has to be seen from a variety of viewpoints (Cohen, 1988).

But, in fact, the care is far from being always optimal, and one of the shortcomings of the deinstitutionalisation policy is the growing number of psychiatric patients who are to be found in institutions for the homeless and in the penal system. An increasing proportion of homeless people in large cities suffer from serious psychiatric illness, primarily chronic psychoses. Homeless people have always been found in such cities, but in recent decades, this population has changed, in quantity, but also in quality, as there are now more women, children, and more people who exhibit serious psychopathology.

Living in the community, the long-term mentally ill are disadvantaged in many ways, besides often having inadequate housing. Shortage of money, social isolation, and having few contacts outside the institution may all add to the obstacles in the way of their social adaptation (Tantam, 1988). These are all factors that, in one respect or another, are part of their 'quality of life', which could, therefore, perhaps be used in the evaluation as a criterion for successful treatment. Unfortunately, though, no unanimously accepted definition exists of the concept. It may be described as a measurement related to the social group, regardless of individual experience, but also as an overall satisfaction with life that can only be determined by the individual (Lau, 1988). In the case of people with chronic psychoses, we are often faced with the problem that the quality of life and social functioning of this group are judged differently by the therapists and by the patients themselves.

Another consequence of deinstitutionalisation is an increasing demand on the relatives. As a result, relatives of the chronically ill frequently voice dissatisfaction with the mental health services and with the professional staff for their lack of support. Many relatives express frankly aggressive feelings towards institutions and various care programmes that have not been able to help the mentally ill sufficiently (Grella & Grusky, 1989; Kuipers *et al*, 1989). An increasing number of relatives are forming groups with the purpose of securing the rights of psychiatric patients, but also to work as pressure groups on the local authorities. Although caring for the long-term mentally ill gives rise to high levels of stress and to a number of burdens, authorities and mental health professionals have not sufficiently recognised this, or taken the burden placed on relatives adequately into consideration, when evaluating the success of community care programmes. Much would be gained if the energy and resources of the professional side and of the patients' network could be joined together.

Treatment strategies

Treatment strategies cannot be discussed in a vacuum. The pattern of care of a chronic psychotic patient is markedly influenced by the country of residence and the social setting, so that a comparison of care provided under different circumstances and with different services available must be related to the different economies concerned (Potthoff *et al*, 1988). The delineation of the patient population at a given time is always a reflection of a number of factors, such as the variety of treatments available outside the psychiatric institution, the quality of primary health care, the attitude of the population towards psychiatric care, and the admission policy of the institution. A good treatment strategy comprises coordinated and structured community services, adequate medication, case management, and comprehensive, accessible services (Lamb, 1989), to mention only a few. Society, however, frequently fails to allocate resources to fulfil these aims, which may result in a large number of the chronically mentally ill being without proper care.

There is no 'right' way to treat the chronically mentally ill, but there are many wrong ways to do so: the choice of treatment is fundamentally an ethical decision (Shaner, 1989). Psychiatrists are daily presented with the difficult problem of deciding what treatment a patient needs and how much good it is likely to do. However, the deinstitutionalisation movement has provided a range of new ways to treat psychiatric illness, and the chronically ill may now receive treatment within various structures of care (Salatini & Elchardus, 1988). But we have to become better at assessing which patients will benefit from which facilities. How can we better prepare patients to leave hospital? Or, in some cases, how can we support chronic patients in their dependency on the asylum (Tantam, 1988)? We have to develop tools that are flexible and useful for all institutions and all cultural settings, for the purpose of describing and comparing the treatment and care of the chronic psychotic population (Potthoff *et al*, 1989). Häfner & an der Heiden (1989) have pointed out that both a monitoring system for mental health care and evaluation of the effectiveness of the new forms of care are urgently needed. We have to set priorities for the values to be applied to care for chronic psychotic patients, and not let ourselves be unduly pressed by non-professional motives. We also have to decide who are going to set these priorities, and thereby influence the treatment strategies. Is it to be the patients, relatives, the mental health professionals, or society at large that in the end has the responsibility for the care of the chronic mentally ill?

References

BURNS, T. P. (1988) The scope and limits of community care. *Current Opinion in Psychiatry*, **1**, 222–225.

COHEN, D. (1988) *Forgotten Millions*. London: Grafton Books.

FREEMAN, H., FRYERS, T. & HENDERSON, J. H. (1985) *Mental Health Services in Europe* (Public Health in Europe Series). Copenhagen: WHO.

GRELLA, C. E. & GRUSKY, O. (1989) Families of the seriously mentally ill and their satisfaction with services. *Hospital and Community Psychiatry*, **40**, 831–835.

HÄFNER, H. (1987) Do we still need beds for psychiatric patients? *Acta Psychiatrica Scandinavica*, **75**, 113–126.

—— & AN DER HEIDEN, W. (1989) The evaluation of mental health care systems. *British Journal of Psychiatry*, **155**, 12–27.

KUIPERS, L., MCCARTHY, B., HURRY, J., *et al.* (1989) Counselling the relatives of the long-term adult mentally ill: II. *British Journal of Psychiatry*, **154**, 775–782.

LAMB, H. L. R. (1989) Improving our public mental health systems. *Archives of General Psychiatry*, **46**, 743–744.

LAU, M. (1988) Livskvalitet hos lungekræftpatienter (Quality of life in lung cancer patients). Doctoral Thesis. Copenhagen: FADL (Association of Danish Medical Students' Publishing Company).

POTTHOFF, P., LEIDE, R., BENDER, W., *et al*, (1988) Time budget analysis for chronic patients. Towards a cost-effectiveness-oriented indicator system for comparing in-patient and out-patient psychiatric care. In *Costs and Effects of Managing Chronic Psychotic Patients* (eds D. Schwefel, *et al*), pp. 228–252. Berlin: Springer.

ROSE, S. M. (1979) Deciphering deinstitutionalization: complexities in policy and program analysis. *Milbank Memorial Fund Quarterly*, **4**, 429–460.

SABATINI, J. & ELCHARDUS, J. M. (1988) Methodological problems of comparing the cost-effectiveness of different mental health institutions. In *Costs and Effects in Managing Chronic Psychotic Patients* (eds D. Schwefel, *et al*), pp. 223–227. Berlin: Springer.

SHANER, A. (1989) Asylums, asphalt and ethics. *Hospital and Community Psychiatry*, **40**, 785–856.

TANTAM, D. (1988) The place of the psychiatric in-patient unit in the care of the chronically psychiatrically ill person. *Current Opinion in Psychiatry*, **1**, 226–231.

3 The establishment, monitoring and evaluation of community care services

C. L. CAZZULLO, G. TACCHINI, CARLO ALTAMURA and MICHELE TANSELLA

In the last two decades, community-based psychiatry has attracted considerable interest, both among professionals and the lay public. In the same period, both in many Western countries and in other parts of the world, a gradual shift has occurred in the organisation of psychiatric services from hospital-centred to community care. In respect of community care, the situation in Italy is unique, both in terms of the speed at which the changes toward a community-based system of psychiatric care have occurred, and also because the nature of the new psychiatric services is prescribed by law. In May 1978, the Italian parliament passed Law 180, the main aims of which were: firstly, to phase out mental hospitals gradually (closing their doors to first admissions after May 1978 and to all admissions after December 1981, but without requiring the rapid discharge of most resident patients); and secondly, to institute a comprehensive and integrated system of psychiatric care in each Unita Locale Socio-Sanitaria (ULSS; local socio-health unit) with between 100 000 and 200 000 inhabitants. Shortly afterwards, Law 180 became part of comprehensive legislation that reformed health services and introduced the Italian National Health Service (NHS).

The major provisions of Law 180 have been extensively reported elsewhere (Tansella & Williams, 1987; Mangen, 1989; Mosher & Burti, 1989); only the main elements, therefore, will be outlined here.

Firstly, the model of community psychiatry proposed in Italy is designed to be an alternative to, rather than to complement, psychiatric hospital-based services (Tansella & Zimmermann-Tansella, 1988). Secondly, the gradual phasing out of mental hospitals, to be achieved by means of a block on admissions, differs considerably from the US community mental health experience, which has been characterised by the relocation of long-stay in-patients to private, non-psychiatric facilities such as nursing homes, boarding-houses, etc. In this latter case, the new community mental health units, financed by public funds, were selecting new populations of patients, rather than serving those discharged from state hospitals (Brown, 1985; Mechanic & Aiken, 1987).

Thirdly, it is hospital psychiatry (with the passage of time increasingly located in general rather than in mental hospitals) which now complements community care, and not vice versa, as in most European programmes for community psychiatry. Finally, integration is sought in Italy between the various psychiatric facilities within the district-based system of care, the same team providing domiciliary, out-patient, and in-patient care – an approach which facilitates continuity of care and a longitudinal perspective on care and support.

Each ULSS is independent administratively, and responsible for the setting up, functioning, and financing of the combined services, including psychiatric care. Both hospital and extramural care are free in public services, but, in addition, there are out-patient and in-patient services, which are defined as '*convenzionati*', i.e. services whose costs are covered by government funds, as well as totally private services whose costs can sometimes be refunded to the user. Various descriptions of the Italian psychiatric reform have appeared in the international literature (e.g. Tranchina *et al*, 1981; De Plato & Minguzzi, 1981; Mosher, 1982, 1983*a*); according to Tansella *et al* (1987), these descriptions can be grouped into three categories:

(a) anecdotal reports of the 'places I have been and people I have met' type
(b) essentially qualitative descriptions, of a documented and in-depth nature, by invited international experts, such as Bennett (1985), and Jablensky & Henderson (1983) on behalf of the World Health Organization
(c) quantitative evaluations of some specific aspects or some particular areas.

However, there is now a need for a more general and integrated evaluation of the actual care system. The present law indicates only in approximate terms the psychiatric services which are to be implemented, and does not contain any explicit functional or organisational obligations. An example can be found in the model proposed by Lombardy Region (1987), but only partially implemented (Fig. 3.1.).

Psychiatric community care in the Milan area

There have been various accounts of the state of implementation of the psychiatric reform in different parts of Italy (De Salvia & Crepet, 1982; Cazzullo *et al*, 1989), and of the gap dividing the 'two Italies', i.e. the north and the south of the country (Scarcella *et al*, 1980). On the other hand, the aim of our work is to use the latest official data published by Lombardy Region (1987), which relate to 1985, to demonstrate the gross inequalities in structure and in distribution of the psychiatric services which exist even

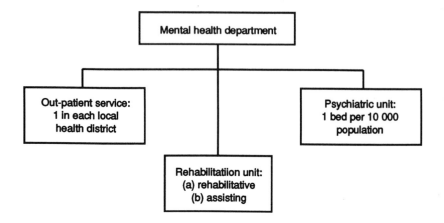

Fig. 3.1. The model of Lombardy region (source: Lombardy Region, 1987)

within a limited geographical area such as the Milan district. This is one
of the most developed and richest parts of the country and, most importantly,
is quite homogeneous and well defined, both culturally and economi-
cally.

Out-patient services (mental health centres (MHC))

The spirit and practice of the psychiatric reform undoubtedly place out-
patient services in a dominant role: the mean values of their components
are shown in Table 3.1, while Table 3.2 indicates the range of variation
for the principal community services. In terms of physical structure, there
are 224.85 m^2 of facilities, with nine rooms on average for the city of Milan,
but in the Lombardy region, this ranges from 30 m^2 in LHD (local health
district) 9 (Busto Arsizio), i.e. only one room, to 931 m^2 in LHD 64 of
Monza; related to the general population, these ratios range from 6.59 to
521.30 m^2 per 100 000 inhabitants. A similar situation is found in relation
to the catchment area, which varies from 28 956 (LHD 75/13) to 120 827
(LHD 75/6) inhabitants in the city of Milan. The variability in terms of
level of activity is even more striking: from 194 patients in actual care in
LHD 75/13, to 1003 in LHD 75/19; from 179 out-patient consultations per
psychiatrist in LHD 75/12, to 1089 in LHD 75/1; from 65 to 626 total home
visits, respectively, in LHDs 75/15 and 75/18. If, on the one hand, there
is a maximum staff of five psychiatrists (LHD 75/19), on the other, it is not
at all exceptional to find a staff comprising one psychiatrist and two nurses
(e.g. LHD 75/2 and 75/7). The same situation applies to psychologists, social
workers, rehabilitation therapists, and aides, as shown in Tables 3.3, 3.4,

TABLE 3.1
Community psychiatric out-patient services in the Milan area

Out-patient services	Mean values of all out-services
Structures	
scheduled	116
area: m^2	225
area per 100 000 population: m^2	15
no. of rooms	9
Existing	90
Population	76 328
No of staff	
psychiatrists	2.45
per 100 000 population	0.16
social workers	1.35
per 100 000 population	0.09
nurses	2.75
per 100 000 population	0.18
No. of patients	458
per 100 000 population	651
No. of visits	
ambulatory	2813
home	1280

TABLE 3.2
Heterogeneity of psychiatric services in Lombardy and in Italy (source: Lombardy Region, 1987)

	Maximum	Minimum
Out-services		
Surface area: m^2	931	30
per 100 000 population	421.3	6.6
Staff	5 psychiatrists	1 psychiatrist
per 100 000 population	5.8	1.7
Patients per 100 000 population	3470	250
Psychiatric units and wards		
Regional beds per 10 000 population	1.35	0.48
	(Regione Trentino)	(Regione Liguria)
Patients admitted per 100 000 population	796	505
Mean stay: days	23.3	4.5
Saturation	188%	21%
Missing	4 local health districts without any unit or ward in Lombardy	
Residential homes		
Beds per 10 000 population	3.4	0.2
	(Sondrio)	(Milan)
Missing	Most local health districts in Lombardy have none	

TABLE 3.3
Out-patient psychiatric services of Milan

Local health district	Population of catchment area	No. of rooms	Area: m²	Patients In charge	1st visits
75/1	106 326	11	200	294	104
75/2	80 181	12	450	434	153
75/3	63 456	9	200	320	63
75/4	76 915	5	140	554	112
75/5	76 994	13	300	419	129
75/6	120 827	14	280	563	200
75/7	36 763	5	86	556	152
75/8	52 593	10	400	300	103
75/9	55 582	8	85	529	98
75/10	101 319	9	160	617	193
75/11	117 700	9	235	639	149
75/12	37 733	4	115	239	59
75/13	28 956	7	126	194	115
75/14	77 564	6	110	453	148
75/15	57 777	8	120	357	94
75/16	55 263	9	240	263	96
75/17	94 239	7	150	522	159
75/18	85 828	5	100	453	166
75/19	105 252	15	400	1003	253
75/20	95 311	15	600	756	163

TABLE 3.4
Out-patient psychiatric services of Milan

Local health district	Ambulatory visits Psychiatrists	Psychologists	Home visits
75/1	1470	1089	588
75/2	4184	570	345
75/3	1191	370	121
75/4	980	334	182
75/5	2137	893	128
75/6	1932	795	119
75/7	1274	258	232
75/8	1856	400	216
75/9	1993	315	414
75/10	1408	728	622
75/11	2740	699	383
75/12	618	179	118
75/13	1068	793	526
75/14	2026	933	235
75/15	2050	630	65
75/16	911	186	95
75/17	3138	692	417
75/18	1472	494	626
75/19	3684	616	477
75/20	5686	1034	545

TABLE 3.5
Out-patient psychiatric services of Milan

Local health district	Psychiatrists	Psychologists	Nurses	Social workers	Aides
75/1	3	1	2	4	4
75/2	1	1	2	2	3
75/3	2	2	2	2	1
75/4	2	1	2	3	1
75/5	4	2	2	3	0
75/6	3	2	2	3	0
75/7	2	3	1	3	1
75/8	2	1	1	3	1
75/9	2	1	1	2	1
75/10	2	1	1	3	1
75/11	3	1	1	3	3
75/12	1	0	0	0	1
75/13	1	1	2	2	0
75/14	2	1	1	5	1
75/15	3	2	2	1	1
75/16	2	1	2	1	1
75/17	3	1	1	2	0
75/18	2	1	1	3	1
75/19	5	2	2	5	1
75/20	4	2	2	5	1

and 3.5. In the last three to four years, in fact, there has been a good deal of staff movement, mainly for career reasons and especially in the less well-established services, but, at present, more than ten years after Law 180, most staff places seem to be in the process of being filled.

Some of the disparities that have been emphasised certainly have specific causes, such as relative inequalities in the socio-economic structure, size of catchment area, therapeutic targets, and working methods of the different teams. However, global differences are so wide and atypical situations so frequent that other factors must be significant. Even the administrative management of the staff is often very diverse: in some LHDs, cars, meal vouchers, and even coats and shoes are provided to personnel, whereas in others, not only are such benefits not available, but there are also complex, time-consuming bureaucratic procedures to obtain authorisation to leave the clinic to visit a patient, and few drugs are available. Even the accessibility of the service is often problematic, e.g. when the clinic is located in a part of the city completely different from the one to be served, as is the case in LHD 75/4. The costs of out-patient services mainly relate to staff, drugs, financial support to patients, and transport, but their amount in any single LHD is not known, nor is it known what percentage of an LHD's total budget is devoted to psychiatric care as a whole. It is almost impossible to obtain such information; perhaps some LHDs do not even calculate it. Furthermore, we are not aware of any study about therapeutic goals, course and outcome of illness, or evaluation of the quality, efficacy, or efficiency of the psychiatric service in any LHD.

On the other hand, it should be noted that almost all the out-patient services in the Milan area were active well before 1978; well-organised professional teams were built up over a considerable time, and had developed therapeutic approaches and goals of their own. Where this occurred, the effects of staff mobility were reduced, but, on the other hand, in some other situations lack of structure and resources prevented any choice of activities, so that the only possibility was simply to care for the most severely ill patients. In other cases, goals were very limited, defined by a 'pragmatism of interventions', which in the end proved reductive: here, therapeutic goals are generated by the interventions themselves, so that the latter become the aim, rather than the tool, of daily practice. Minor psychiatric disturbances such as neuroses and psychosomatic disorders are seldom, if at all, treated in the out-patient services, particularly in urban areas, with some specific exceptions such as LHD 75/7, where the resident population is generally older and more stable. Almost everywhere, however, relationships with general practitioners are quite limited.

Hospital psychiatric units (diagnosis and care units)

Table 3.6 shows the mean values of the principal features of diagnosis and care units (D&Cs) in Milan and Lombardy region. These are located within general hospitals and have a maximum of 15 beds for each operative unit (OU), but, at least in some regions, the same D&C can include several OUs; each OU serves two or three LHDs. Most D&Cs have three beds per room and occupy more than 500 m^2, though there are exceptions: for instance, 350 m^2 and 30 beds in Como (OU 4), i.e. 11 m^2 per bed, as against 55 m^2 at Niguarda Hospital, Milan (OU 36 and 37), the OUs occupying a total of 1000 m^2. Some D&Cs (Gallarate and Merate) are still only just being completed, more than ten years after Law 180 was passed.

The mean catchment area has 236 637 inhabitants, but the range is from 55 881 in Gavardo (OU 12) to 377 214 at San Carlo Hospital in Milan (OU 42). Relating the number of beds to population, we find a mean value of 7.80 beds per 100 000 inhabitants, with a minimum of only 3.18 and a maximum of 26.79 at San Carlo Hospital and in Gavardo, respectively. Medical staff mostly share their time between the out-patient services and the D&C; the Chief of Service also has responsibility for the activities of the LHDs pertaining to his or her unit, i.e. of the whole OU. The biggest and most renowned hospitals, such as Niguarda and the Polyclinic in Milan, have a national competence as Scientific Institutes of Research and Care,

TABLE 3.6
Psychiatric wards in the Milan area

General hospital psychiatric wards	Mean values
Structures	
in Milan	8
no. of beds	119
area: m^2	569
in the outskirts	10
no. of beds	145
area: m^2	503
No. of beds per 100 000 population	
in Milan	7.80
in the outskirts	9.50
No. of staff	
psychiatrists	3
director	1
chief of service	1
nurses	16
No. of in-patients per 100 000 population	1596
No. of admissions	29
Length of stay: days	12.04
Occupancy level: percentage of maximum	85.37
Percentage of patients undergoing compulsory treatment	19.63
Percentage of patients who are new admissions	55

are directly administered by the Ministry of Health, and can also admit patients from districts other than their own. They can also employ a staff independent of the LHDs whose duties, besides in-patient care, comprise medical research, counselling, out-patient care, and teaching – if a university medical school is attached.

The practice of admitting psychiatric patients to other units, usually general medical ones, is fairly uncommon in Lombardy, though common in other regions, e.g. Emilia-Romagna: thus, data about admissions in Lombardy are quite reliable. The number of in-patients in the city of Milan ranges from a minimum of 505.07 (OU 40) to a maximum of 796.43 per 100 000 population (OU 39); the number of admissions is between 54.45 (OU 40) and 209.10 per 100 000 population (OU 35). Mean hospital stay is 12.04 days and ranges from a minimum of 4.57 (OU 25, Monza) to a maximum of 23.26 days (OU 39 at the Polyclinic Hospital in Milan); the maximum occupancy recorded in 1985 was 188.49% in OU 51 (Cremona), while the minimum was 21.05% in OU 21 (Melegnano). In this respect also, the values are widely spread around the mean: indices of occupancy greater than 100%, mainly through the use of beds on wheels, are not unusual and bear witness to the overcrowded conditions in the psychiatric units.

Patients admitted were already known to the hospital unit in 45% of cases; the most severe of them were under compulsory treatment, with a maximum ratio of 37.88 at OU 14 (Brescia), and a minimum of 4.14 at OU 28 (Garbagnate).

Occupancy indices and readmission percentages point to the fact that the actual work of hospital units is often affected by the pressure of admitting new patients under compulsory treatments which cannot be delayed, as well as others who may have been waiting for a relatively long time. Average waiting times before admission are not known, but it is evident that a hospital unit can be regarded as a filter, where non-dischargeable patients can accumulate and occupy some beds for many months. Such patients suffer greatly from the severe lack of residential homes and rehabilitation units specifically designed for their condition.

Data from the Regional Authority do not include the 'out-of-district' patients: the rule is that every psychiatric patient has to be admitted to the psychiatric unit of the LHD where he or she lives, and, as a consequence, patients are transferred as soon as possible to their own in-patient service. However, this is not always feasible, as, for instance, in the case of foreigners; only some of the bigger hospitals are allowed to admit such patients, and this is why the data about some D&Cs are underestimates.

No data are available about the *convenzionati* private clinics; in Milan and the Lombardy region, there are four with a total of 420 beds, as compared with the 615 beds in all the D&Cs; from a qualitative point of view, their activity is very similar to that of the D&Cs, while, quantitatively, it has been estimated that they have about 3700 admissions per year, as against 11 854 in the public services.

In-patient care is usually both pharmacological and psychotherapeutic, or else purely pharmacological; when possible, therapeutic continuity is preserved; i.e., the same psychiatrist that saw a patient in the out-patient facility cares for him in the hospital unit. If that is not possible, a discharge programme is usually agreed upon with the out-patient service team. Quality, efficacy, or efficiency studies about D&Cs or out-patient services have not been carried out in Lombardy. Similarly, the running costs of the individual units are unknown.

Intermediate residential facilities

Data from the 'intermediate residential facilities' (IRF) are displayed in Table 3.7: they are residential homes or communities where nursing care is provided either daily or more sporadically, but seldom at night. In addition to full-time residence, patients can use them only partially, e.g. at night or during the day. In Milan, these facilities are concentrated in only two of the 20 LHDs of the city (LHDs 75/6 and 75/8), and they, respectively, occupy 270 m^2 with 10 rooms and 400 m^2 with 13 rooms. There are also

TABLE 3.7
Psychiatric residential facilities in the Milan area

Services	Mean values
Intermediate residential centres: both night and day hospital	
in Milan	2
no. of beds	17
in the outskirts	14
no. of beds	50
no. of beds per 100 000 population	0.89
area: m^2	335
no. of rooms per centre	11
no. of patients per room	3
Independent day hospitals (open 3–5 days a week)	12
no. of rooms per hospital	4
Rehabilitation units:	
scheduled	56
existing	0
Long-stay institutions	4
no. of beds per institution	475
length of stay: days	312

12 day hospitals which are independent of the rest of the community services; their organisational and administrative status is still provisional, after more than ten years.

The facility devoted to medium-term and long-term admissions, both with therapeutic and caring goals, is the residential therapeutic centre (RTC), serving 158 000 inhabitants, i.e. approximately one for each LHD and more than one for each D&C. These should have between 12 and 20 beds and function as day hospitals, night hospitals, or out-patient centres; however, of 56 scheduled and approved RTCs, none is yet operating. Finally, there are four *convenzionati* private institutions for long-term admissions, with a total of 1900 beds, 475 each on average: in 1985, they had 2230 admissions, with a mean stay of 312 days. In order to meet the criteria of Law 180, these are mostly converting themselves into groupings of therapeutic communities of 20–30 patients, each with an independent staff and specific rehabilitative and resocialisation programmes. This is one of the reasons that waiting times for admission to them have become longer and longer, at present amounting to several months. The most severely ill patients therefore have no alternative but to spend these months in D&Cs, but, to satisfy the request for new admissions, severely ill patients often have to be discharged, thus transferring the burden to their families and to out-patient services. This is one of the factors that led to the setting up of relatives' associations in Italy, especially in the cities.

Conclusions

The heterogeneity and inequalities of individual facilities in Lombardy are so great that psychiatric epidemiologists have sometimes felt lost and

40   *Cazzullo* et al

impotent (Lombardy Region, 1987; Cazzullo *et al*, 1989). Our impression, which certainly does not apply to psychiatry alone, is that the individual LHDs have become many small, independent health republics, where therapeutic work is not really aimed at clinical goals, because of the limitations of what is feasible. This is the case even when referring to a geographical area that, compared with the rest of the country, is relatively homogeneous and wealthy. The efforts of psychiatric workers and patients' relatives have not been sufficiently strong to overcome present inadequacies or to accelerate the decisions of administrative and political authorities about these problems.

Monitoring psychiatric care in South Verona (1979–88)

South Verona is an area in northern Italy with 75 000 inhabitants, where a new, community-based system of care, the South Verona Community Psychiatric Service (CPS), has operated since 1978. This system, which is based on the provisions of the Italian psychiatric reform, is alternative to the old, hospital-centred system, providing care and support to all types of patients, without back-up from the mental hospital, where only a few long-stay in-patients continue to reside. Details on the organisation and provision of the South Verona CPS have been published elsewhere (Burti *et al*, 1986; Tansella *et al*, 1991). However, the literature so far contains only scanty evidence on monitoring and evaluating the comprehensive care provided by community psychiatric services in defined areas over a long period of time.

The South Verona Psychiatric Case Register (PCR), which started on 31 December 1978, covers all psychiatric hospitals and units (including private hospitals) of the province of Verona, as well as out-patient and day-patient facilities located in the same area. Contacts of adult South Verona residents with psychiatrists, psychologists, social workers, and psychiatric nurses are routinely recorded (Tansella *et al*, 1991).

Trends in the provision of psychiatric care in the period 1979–88 have been analysed with the South Verona PCR. Both one-day and one-year prevalence figures and incidence rates are lower than in other register areas outside Italy, partly because of the smaller number of specialised, out-patient services available in South Verona, and partly because of less use of in-patient care in the area. Moreover, there is a tendency in Italy to care for elderly patients in geriatric institutions, which are outside the psychiatric system.

Most of the patients seen in any year are treated without in-patient care: this applies to all diagnostic groups except affective psychosis. Rates of compulsory admission dropped dramatically after the reform. Although the total number of admissions to all in-patient psychiatric facilities (including private hospitals) in 1988 was only 8.4% lower than that found in 1977 (one year prior to the reform), the mean number of occupied beds in 1988 was 47% lower than in 1977 (Tansella *et al*, 1991).

In South Verona the point-prevalence of long-stay in-patients (those patients in hospital – both public and private – on census day who have been there continuously for the previous 365 days or longer) has slowly decreased over the years, and there is a negligible build-up of new long-stay in-patients. The South Verona CPS is now taking care of most psychiatric patients who, before the reform, would have been admitted to the mental hospital and become long-stay patients. These patients, who may be defined as long-term (chronic) patients in the community, have consistently accumulated since 1981, and are making intensive use of psychiatric community services. In the South Verona PCR, they have been defined as those patients, not long-stay hospital residents, who have remained in contact with some form of psychiatric service, without a break of 91 days or more between contacts.

Chronic psychiatric patients in the community were identified from the PCR over six years following the reform. Six first-contact socio-demographic variables (sex, age, marital status, living situation, education, occupational status) and two clinical variables (ICD–9 diagnosis and past history of state psychiatric hospital admission) were studied for these patients.

Four full cohort-years of post-reform chronic patients were followed for a two-year period to determine their subsequent patterns of care. Log-linear analysis was used to examine the interaction of cohort-year with outcome, and the above socio-demographic and clinical variables were studied both individually and in combination. It was found that 36.4% of post-reform community chronic patients remained in long-term contact with psychiatric services for two years after they were first identified. Logistic analysis revealed that none of the socio-demographic and clinical variables studied, individually or in combination, were predictive of the probability of remaining in long-term contact with community psychiatric services (Viscogliosi-Calabrese *et al*, 1991).

Previous studies in the area (Balestrieri *et al*, 1987) showed that 88% of those patients who had become long-stay in-patients in state psychiatric hospitals (pre-reform hospital chronic patients) remained long-stay during the next two years. The clinical and social implications of accumulating chronic patients in the community after the psychiatric reform, rather than long-stay in-patients in state psychiatric hospitals, need to be considered. The present results, if confirmed, would suggest that long-term community care by the South Verona Community Psychiatric Service induces less service dependence and chronic use than did the old hospital-based system of care.

A retrospective follow-up study on a cohort of schizophrenic patients

A retrospective follow-up study was conducted on the full cohort of those South Verona residents who, in 1979, contacted the psychiatric services monitored by the PCR and received an ICD–9 diagnosis of 'schizophrenic or other functional non-affective psychosis'. The 60 patients who met the inclusion criteria were traced in 1986 and interviewed, the researchers using standardised instruments (PSE–9, DAS–2, PIRS). Patients living in the community were found to be in a variety of living conditions, but none who were judged to need support were without it (i.e. none were *abbandonati*), including those who were out of contact with psychiatric services. An excess mortality was found, within the two-fold increase reported in other studies: only one death was due to suicide.

Comparisons between patients who remained in the mental hospital and community patients revealed that the clinical condition of mental hospital patients tended to remain unchanged through the years, while their social skills declined. These patients were withdrawn, unable to relate to others, and had no interests or activities. On the other hand, community patients were most frequently disturbed in their occupational role and heterosexual role behaviour. Symptoms in community patients correlated with social performance, but not consistently (Mignolli *et al*, 1991).

The results of this study underline the likelihood that prolonged contact with psychiatric services, even if community-orientated, does not in itself entirely prevent social disability. A parallel study was conducted on the same cohort of patients, using a procedure recently developed by Brewin *et al* (1987) for assessing the needs for care of long-term mentally ill patients in the community (Needs for Care Assessment Schedule (NFCAS)). It was found that the South Verona CPS was meeting both the clinical and living skills needs of its patients. On the other hand, the patients in contact with other services or private practitioners were presenting few problems, and those out of contact with any form of service were presenting the lowest number of problems. It was found that in its present form, the NFCAS is not appropriate for rating long-stay in-patients still living in Italian mental hospitals (Lesage *et al*, 1991).

Conclusion

According to the Italian model, community-based psychiatry may be defined as a system of care devoted to a defined population and based on a comprehensive and integrated mental health service. Such a service should include a wide spectrum of out-patient, day-patient, and general hospital in-patient services, as well as both staffed and unstaffed residential facilities. It should ensure multidisciplinary team work, early diagnosis, prompt treatment, continuity of care, social support, and close liaison with other community medical and social services, in particular with general practitioners (Tansella, 1986). According to this definition, the mental hospital is intended to be gradually superseded and finally closed. To what extent this model has been implemented in Italy since 1978 remains unclear (Crepet, 1990). The available data show that there is a marked regional inequality in the provision of services (Tansella & Williams, 1987; Bollini *et al*, 1988), but recent data indicate that 32% of Italian community psychiatric services were defined as comprehensive and integrated, and comparable to those in South Verona (Frisanco, 1989).

Ten years' experience in South Verona has confirmed that it is possible to deal with the full spectrum of psychiatric morbidity within a community-based alternative service, with limited back-up from the mental hospital, where only 18 old, long-stay in-patients from South Verona continue to reside (on 31 December 1989). The mental hospital has now been closed to new admissions for 12 years and to all admissions for eight years (Tansella, 1991).

Further research is necessary to evaluate the clinical and social outcome in different groups of patients and to explore fully the question of whether the handicaps of people with severe and long-term disabilities have been significantly reduced and their quality of life enhanced by the South Verona community-based system of care.

Acknowledgements

The studies in South Verona reported in this chapter were supported by the Consiglio Nazionale delle Recerche (CNR Roma), by Progetto Finalizzato Medicina Preventiva e Riabilitativa 1982–1987 through contracts to Professor M. Tansella, and by the Regione Veneto, Ricerca Sanitaria Finalizzata (contracts no. 77.03.85 and no. 134.03.86).

References

BALESTRIERI, M., MICCIOLO, R. & TANSELLA, M. (1987) Long-stay and long-term psychiatric patients in an area with a community-based system of care. A register follow-up study. *International Journal of Social Psychiatry*, **33**, 251–262.

BENNETT, D. H. (1985) The changing pattern of mental health care in Trieste. *International Journal of Mental Health*, **14**, 70–92.

BOLLINI, P., REICH, M. & MUSCETTOLA, G. (1988) Revision of the Italian psychiatric reform: North/South differences and future strategies. *Social Science and Medicine*, **12**, 1327–1335.

BREWIN, C. R., WING, J. K., MANGEN, S. P., *et al* (1987) Principles and practice of measuring needs in the long-term mentally ill: the MRC Needs for Care Assessment. *Psychological Medicine*, **17**, 971–981.

BROWN, P. (1985) *The Transfer of Care: Psychiatric Deinstitutionalization and its Aftermath*. Henley-on-Thames: Routledge & Kegan Paul.

BURTI, L., GARZOTTO, N., SICILIANI, O., *et al* (1986) South Verona psychiatric service: an integrated system of community care. *Hospital and Community Psychiatry*, **37**, 809–813.

CAZZULLO, C. L., COPPOLA, M. T. & TACCHINI, G. (1989) La Psychiatrie en Italie: situation actuelle et perspectives d'avenir. *Psychiatrie Française*, **1**, 29–44.

CREPET, P. (1990) A transition period in psychiatric care in Italy ten years after the reform. *British Journal of Psychiatry*, **156**, 27–36.

DE PLATO, G. & MINGUZZI, G. (1981) A short history of psychiatric renewal in Italy. *Psychiatry and Social Science*, **1**, 71–77.

DE SALVIA, D. & CREPET, P. (1982) *Psichiatria senza Manicomio: Epidemiologia Critica della Riforma*. Milano: Feltrinelli.

FRISANCO, R. (1989) The quality of psychiatric care since the reform law: the "CENSIS survey". *International Journal of Social Psychiatry*, **35**, 81–89.

JABLENSKY, A. & HENDERSON, J. (1983) Report on a visit to the South Verona Community Psychiatric Service. WHO Assignment Report. Geneva and Copenhagen: WHO.

LESAGE, A. D., MIGNOLLI, G., FACCINCANI, C., et al (1991) Standardised assessment of the needs for care in a cohort of patients with schizophrenic psychoses. In *Community-based Psychiatry: Long-term Patterns of Care in South Verona* (ed. M. Tansella), Psychological Medicine Monograph (suppl. 19), pp. 27–33. Cambridge: Cambridge University Press.

LOMBARDY REGION (1985) Psichiatria, Neuropsichiatria Infantile, Epilessia. *Notizie Sanita'*, 11, 83–154.

—— (1987) *Incontri di psichiatria, Assessorato al coordinamento per i servizi sociali.* Regione Lombardia.

MANGEN, S. (ed.) (1989) The Italian psychiatric experience: the first ten years. Special issue of *International Journal of Social Psychiatry*, 35, 1–127.

MECHANIC, D. & AIKEN, L. H. (1987) Improving the care of patients with chronic mental illness. *New England Journal of Medicine*, 317, 1634–1638.

MIGNOLLI, G., FACCINCANI, C. & PLATT, (1991) Psychopathology and social performance in a cohort of patients with schizophrenic psychoses. A seven-year follow-up study. In *Community-based Psychiatry: Long-term Patterns of Care in South Verona* (ed. B. Tansella), Psychological Medicine Monograph (suppl. 19), pp. 17–26. Cambridge: Cambridge University Press.

MOSHER, L. (1982) Italy's revolutionary mental health law: an assessment. *American Journal of Psychiatry*, 139, 199–203, 198.

—— (1983a) Radical deinstitutionalization: the Italian experience. *International Journal of Mental Health*, 11, 129–136.

—— (1983b) Recent developments in the care, treatment, and rehabilitation of the chronic mentally ill in Italy. *Hospital and Community Psychiatry*, 34, 947–950.

—— & BURTI, L. (1989) *Community Mental Health: Principles and Practice.* New York: Norton.

SCARCELLA, M., MACRI, V., BISIGNANI, A., et al (1980) *Pericoloso a Se' e agli Altri.* Bari: De Donato.

TANSELLA, M. (1986) Community psychiatry without mental hospitals. The Italian experience: a review. *Journal of the Royal Society of Medicine*, 79, 664–669.

—— (ed.) (1991) *Community-based Psychiatry: Long-term Patterns of Care in South Verona.* Psychological Medicine Monograph Supplement. Cambridge: Cambridge University Press (in press).

——, DE SALVIA, D. & WILLIAMS, P. (1987) The Italian psychiatric reform: some quantitative evidence. *Social Psychiatry*, 22, 37–48.

—— & WILLIAMS, P. (1987) The Italian experience and its implications. *Psychological Medicine*, 17, 283–289.

—— & ZIMMERMANN-TANSELLA, CH. (1988) From mental hospitals to alternative community services. In *Modern Perspectives in Clinical Psychiatry* (ed. J. G. Howells), pp. 130–148. New York: Brunner/Mazel.

——, BALESTRIERI, M., MENEGHELLI, G., et al (1991) Trends in the provision of psychiatric care 1979–1988. In *Community-based Psychiatry: Long-term Patterns of Care in South Verona* (ed. M. Tansella). Psychological Medicine Monograph Supplement. Cambridge: Cambridge University Press (in press).

TRANCHINA, P., ARCHI, G. & FERRARA, G. (1981) The new legislation in Italian psychiatry. *International Journal of Law and Psychiatry*, 4, 181–190.

VISCOGLIOSI-CALABRESE, L., MICCIOLO, R. & TANSELLA, M. (1991) Patterns of care for chronic patients after the Italian psychiatric reform: a longitudinal case-register study. *Social Science and Medicine* (in press).

4 Services for patients with chronic mental illness: results of research and experience

JOHN SHANKS

Provision for people with chronic severe psychiatric illness is the major challenge facing mental illness services in many different countries at present. The House of Commons Social Services Select Committee on Community Care (1985) pointed out that the real test of a service is not whether it provides adequately for those who least require it, but whether it provides well for those who need it most.

The current situation

In a recent UK survey, the National Unit for Psychiatric Research and Development found that 40% of District Health Authorities have, in practical terms, no services outside hospital dedicated to this most vulnerable group, while 54% have no system to monitor the continuity of care they give. However, the growing specialty of psychiatric rehabilitation does mean that in many Districts, there is now a consultant psychiatrist with a particular remit to provide service to people with persistent disability resulting from mental illness. Practice varies considerably in respect of how much time is devoted to patients already in the community, as opposed to those in hospital, and also as to whether or not other parts of the mental illness service take any responsibility for the continuing care of people with chronic problems.

In 1981, the Department of Health and Social Security established the beginnings of what is now a network of 11 National Demonstration Services in Psychiatric Rehabilitation. Services which are designated in this way have been assessed by a multidisciplinary team of their peers as exemplifying some aspect of good practice in the rehabilitation of people with psychiatric illness. The intention is that a National Demonstration Service should provide a focus for the dissemination of good practice to other services, encouraging them to improve and develop their own practice.

The transition to the community

Evidence from the USA, and more recently from the UK, suggests that the transition from an institution-based to a locally based service is often accompanied by a drift of resources. The focus of the service tends to move away from people with the most severe disabilities, such as chronic schizophrenia, towards a less severely disabled group of clients, which may include people with anxiety, depression, and relationship difficulties – sometimes dismissively described as the 'worried well' but more accurately characterised as suffering from non-psychotic, psychiatric morbidity. This drift is rarely intentional, and often goes unnoticed until it is revealed by monitoring or research. The reasons for it are many, but may include the tendency of some community services to rely too heavily on the patients' own ability to seek help. This will tend to equate demand for care with need for care, and to select clients in favour of the more perceptive and articulate. However, drift is not an inevitable consequence of the transition to the community; it is quite possible for a community-based service to make a priority of people with chronic mental illness, but this requires a clear setting of goals and monitoring of their achievement. Of course, people with anxiety and depression have real needs too, but there is a greater range of options to meet these needs, such as primary care services, self-help, voluntary groups, and social services. People disabled by chronic severe psychiatric illness have few options other than specialist mental health services.

The most rational use of health service resources would be that primary care services should themselves manage a greater proportion than at present of people presenting with relatively minor forms of psychiatric morbidity. This would leave specialist mental health services free to concentrate on the needs of those with the more severe forms of psychiatric illness. A number of studies have looked at patients discharged from hospital, often after many years of residence, to life in the community, and three of them are described here.

The Friern/Claybury study

Both Friern Barnet and Claybury are large mental hospitals which are scheduled for closure in the near future; patients resident for many years in these hospitals are being resettled in locally based facilities.

The Department of Health and the Regional Health Authority took the opportunity to commission research (in the TAPS project) on the relative costs of hospital care and community care for matched groups of patients. In one sample, for all of the 25 patients in the community group, the cost of care was less than that for patients still resident in hospital. The savings from placement in the community were greatest for the less severely disabled individuals in the study. Since the patients who still remain in hospital include some of the most severely disabled, it may well be that for some of these most dependent people, the cost of care in the community will be greater than the cost of care in hospital (Knapp *et al*, 1987; see also Leff, Chapter 7).

The PSSRU study

This study looked at those projects which were set up following a Department of Health and Social Security circular on care in the community, and it included both mentally ill and mentally handicapped people (DHSS, 1983). A number of findings were particularly striking; firstly, no client lost contact with services, became destitute or homeless, or was imprisoned after leaving hospital. There were very few readmissions to hospital and most of these were short term. It is interesting to speculate what it was about these projects which allowed them to avoid the problems which have sometimes attended placement of institutional residents in the community. The study strongly implies that proper case management was vitally important in maintaining adequate follow-up and in protecting clients from gaps in the provision of service.

Both the costs and the benefits of community placement were examined. One benefit was that most of the clients expressed a preference for community placement over previous hospital residence. In terms of outcome, mentally handicapped people showed signs of an increase in skills, abilities, or symptoms. Compared with the cost of hospital care, care in the community was less expensive for the mentally ill clients in the project, but more expensive for the mentally handicapped. In view of the results of the Friern/Claybury study, this may represent the effect of the *severity* rather than the *type* of disability, since within the projects examined the mentally handicapped clients were generally more severely disabled than the mentally ill. For all groups of clients, more severe disability means higher costs, whether in hospital or in the community. There was a tremendous variation in the cost of care among different community projects; this variation was much greater than the variation between different hospitals. Voluntary sector projects came out better than either NHS or local authority facilities in terms of cost-effectiveness – a finding which may well repay further study (Knapp & Beecham, 1989).

The Douglas House study

This study took as its subject a group of 22 patients with chronic severe psychiatric illness, all of whom were judged still to require 24-hour nursing care after more than six months' in-patient stay. The patients were randomly allocated to two different patterns of care: routine care in a district general hospital (DGH) psychiatric unit or care in a hostel ward (Douglas House). The hostel ward aims to offer the 24-hour staffing which is characteristic of hospital units, but in a more domestic setting, with a higher staff–patient ratio, and with patients taking more responsibility for their own care.

The two patterns of care were compared on both costs and benefits: the hostel ward emerged as superior to the DGH unit in both respects. Compared to DGH residents, Douglas House residents acquired more domestic skills, made more use of community facilities, displayed less psychotic impairment, and experienced less harassment and victimisation from other residents. Douglas House residents preferred the environment of the hostel ward to the DGH unit. The time course over which these benefits accrued is interesting in itself; over the three-year course of the study, it seemed that DGH residents continued to accumulate disability, mainly because of their psychotic impairment, while hostel ward residents maintained their level of ability. The hostel ward was also significantly less expensive overall. Although the higher than usual staff ratio involved a greater expenditure on nursing care, this was more than offset by savings on support services such as catering and domestic staff, since in the hostel ward, patients themselves perform these activities as part of the daily routine (Hyde *et al*, 1987).

Destitute homeless people with mental illness

The sight of homeless people huddled under arches in some inner cities is a familiar one, and a number of studies have confirmed what appearances suggest – that a considerable proportion suffer from schizophrenia and other serious psychiatric illnesses, 20–50% in many studies (Timms & Fry, 1989). Most are not receiving any treatment for their illness; typically, they have been in contact with mental health services in the past, but have dropped out of care through failure to attend for day-care or out-patient appointments. There may be very real practical difficulties of access to health services for people who do not have a settled way of life, but a problem of acceptability of services also exists. Priest (1975) noted in his study of residents of common lodging-houses in Edinburgh that "the typical lodging-house resident does not choose to seek treatment for his psychiatric morbidity". Service providers and planners need to ask themselves what it is about the current pattern of services that makes homeless people so apparently reluctant to seek help from them. The Department of Health has consulted voluntary organisations in this field to consider how a better service might be provided to this needy group and how a clearer picture of their requirements and preferences might be obtained.

An initiative was announced on 12 July 1990 by Stephen Dorrell, Parliamentary Under-Secretary of State for Health. This programme will offer accommodation and psychiatric care to homeless people in Central London who are mentally ill. The scheme is likely to cost more than £5 million over two years. It includes the provision of 60 new short-term hostel places with social support, and new community-based psychiatric teams in three of the Thames Regions. The aim is first to contact and then help homeless, mentally ill people and to provide up to 450 new housing places to which residents of the short-term hostels can progress. The community psychiatric teams are designed around the successful model of the Psychiatric Team for the Single Homeless which has been piloted and evaluated by Dr Philip Timms and his colleagues at Guy's Hospital.

Health and social services authorities in Central London are being asked to work, together with appropriate voluntary organisations, to make a fuller assessment of the numbers of homeless, mentally ill people and to identify how their health and social care needs are best met. The initiative will be evaluated and the results should provide useful information for other parts of the country.

The need for asylum

It is now clear that in every District there will be some patients who require long-term care and supervision of a type which is usually found only in hospital. Data from the Worcester Development Project suggests that in a small town like Kidderminster, this amounts to about seven patients per 100 000 population, of whom many suffer from organic brain disorders, while information from inner-city districts, such as Camberwell, suggests a higher incidence, of 20 patients per 100 000 (Garety *et al*, 1988), of whom the majority suffer from schizophrenia.

The challenge for services is to provide the asylum which these patients need without the undesirable features of the traditional large mental hospital – 'asylum without asylums'. Hospital hostels have emerged as one possible solution to this problem. Although there is no standard model, all of them attempt to provide high levels of care and supervision in a setting which is more domestic than a hospital unit. A number have been subject to evaluation, such as Douglas House, already described, and the Department has published a report setting out the most important findings from the current network of hospital hostels (Young, 1991).

An interesting development in the provision of day care and work opportunities has been the 'clubhouse' model, pioneered at Fountain House in New York, and now reproduced in a number of other countries. Mentally ill people become members of a social club, which revolves around the provision of the usual range of amenities that club members expect. Social contact, meals, refreshments, and entertainment are organised by club members themselves for the benefit of all, and these provide a range of employment opportunities within the club itself. In addition, many clubhouses have managed to obtain work placements in open employment by offering employers the guarantee that the post will always be filled. If a club member is unable to go to work because of illness, then the post will be filled temporarily by another club member or by a staff member. The important difference from conventional day-care centres is the explicit recognition of mentally ill people as a resource in themselves, not merely recipients of care. It is perhaps this which accounts for the sense of belonging to something worthwhile, which is very evident in members of USA clubhouses. A London-based voluntary organisation opened the first British clubhouse in 1991.

Future developments

Care programmes

Health authorities have recently received central advice that they must, by 1991, establish care programmes to ensure the delivery of adequate services to people disabled by chronic severe mental illness (Department of Health, 1990a). More detailed guidance will follow. Much experience has now been accumulated by services which have made it a priority to focus on people with chronic severe disabilities: such services have clearly pointed out the value of a proper system of case management. While there are differences among services in nomenclature and in the precise allocation of tasks among individuals, a number of features of case management are common to all, and may therefore be the essential requirement.

Firstly, we need an information system (such as a register) to ensure that patients can be identified for follow-up and to prevent patients from losing touch with the service by failing to attend for appointments. Personal computers have made it much easier to establish and maintain such a database.

Secondly, we need case management which encompasses both administrative and therapeutic functions. The task of ensuring that services provided from different sources amount to a package which efficiently meets the patient's identified needs demands essentially administrative skills of communication, coordination, and negotiation with the providers of service. In addition, staff in direct contact with patients and their carers have to act as the channel for communication between patients and all those involved in their care. Some services have divided the two functions between an administrator with the title of 'case manager', and a therapist who is identified as 'key worker'. Other services combine the two tasks in one person, under the title of 'case manager'. However, the important requirement is that both functions should actually be carried out. Evidence is now beginning to accumulate that mental health services which introduce an effective case management system experience a reduction in usage of hospital resources and an increased uptake of community resources (Shepherd, 1990).

RCPsych guidance on discharge procedures

In London, in 1984, a mentally ill woman (Sharon Campbell) killed her social worker. The subsequent inquiry (the Spokes report) considered the provision of care to people with chronic mental illness, and made a number of recommendations. One of these was that the Royal College of Psychiatrists draw up guidelines on the procedures which should be followed to ensure adequate follow-up for a mentally ill person being discharged from hospital. The College has accepted this task and will be consulting with the other professions involved in providing mental health care to produce what will be in effect a statement of minimum acceptable standards of practice for discharge and follow-up.

Community care reforms

In 1987, the then Secretary of State for Social Services, Norman Fowler, requested Sir Roy Griffiths to consider the arrangements for delivery of community care with a view to producing recommendations on the most effective use of public funds. In 1988, Sir Roy produced his report, *Community Care – Agenda for Action*, which made a number of recommendations on how the current system might be improved. In July 1989, the then Secretary of State for Health, Kenneth Clarke, announced that the Government accepted the principal recommendations of the Griffiths Report, and set out proposals in the White Paper *Caring for People* (UK Government, 1989*a*). There will be major changes in the way in which social care for mentally ill people is funded. Local authority social services departments will be given the responsibility of allocating a new unified source of funding for social care services on the basis of assessments of individual need.

A new specific grant is directed at encouraging local authorities to make their necessary contribution to services, in line with health authority plans and objectives. This grant will be payable by health authorities on the basis of plans put to them by the relevant local authorities (Department of Health, 1990*b*).

NHS reforms

The White Paper *Working for Patients*, which announced fundamental changes in the workings of the National Health Service, was criticised in some circles for not attending more specifically to mental health and other community services (UK Government, 1989*b*). This document was concerned with setting out broad principles which would apply across the whole of the NHS, and thus it is not surprising that little attempt was made to differentiate

C

between specialties. However, the implications of the NHS review are as important for mental health services as for any other sector. The explicit separation of the roles of purchaser and provider of health care services is a direct parallel to the similar separation from social care services proposed in the companion document *Caring for People*. In both cases, the intention is to widen the range of options available to those who use the service, and to make the best use of available resources.

The initial contracts between purchasers and providers are likely to be relatively simple block contracts, which specify access to a defined range of facilities and reflect existing patterns of service use. But, even at this early stage, purchasers will need to have some way of specifying and monitoring the quality of the service provided, as well as the volume. The definition and measurement of quality in mental health services is still at an early stage of development. This monitoring requirement therefore represents a major challenge to the mental health services to identify ways of measuring outcome and other parameters relevant to quality (Jenkins, 1990).

Conclusions

The provision of good care to those severely disabled by chronic psychiatric illness requires long-term planning and is likely to involve changing contributions from a number of different agencies. Since the organisational demands are high, and signs of improvement in clients may be hard to see, it is not surprising that such a complex task has sometimes gone by default. However, it is an area of care which has also produced some of the most ingenious and encouraging developments in service provision, and it is one which is likely to continue to grow.

Acknowledgement

This paper is Crown Copyright. The views are those of the author and do not necessarily reflect Department of Health Policy.

References

DEPARTMENT OF HEALTH (1990a) *The Care Programme Approach for People with a Mental Illness Referred to the Specialist Psychiatric Services.* Circular HC (90)23/LASSL(90)11. London: Department of Health.
——— (1990b) *Specific Grant for the Development of Social Care Services for People with a Mental Illness.* Circular HC(90)24/LAC(90)10. London: Department of Health.
DEPARTMENT OF HEALTH AND SOCIAL SECURITY (1983) *Care in the Community.* HC(83)6 LAC(83)5. London: HMSO.

GARETY, P. A., AFELE, H. K. & ISAACS, A. D. (1988) A hostel ward for new long-stay psychiatric patients: the careers of the first 10 years' residents. *Bulletin of the Royal College of Psychiatrists*, **12**, 183–186.

HOUSE OF COMMONS (1985) *Second Paper from the Social Services Select Committee Session 1984–1985. Community Care with Special Reference to Adult Mentally Ill and Mentally Handicapped People.* London: HMSO.

HYDE, C., BRIDGES, K., GOLDBERG, D., *et al* (1987) The evaluation of a hostel ward: a controlled study using modified cost-benefit analysis. *British Journal of Psychiatry*, **151**, 805–812.

JENKINS, R. (1990) Towards a system of outcome: indicators for mental health. *British Journal of Psychiatry*, **157**, 500–515.

KNAPP, M., BEECHAM, J. & RENSHAW, J. (1987) The cost-effectiveness of psychiatric reprovision services. Discussion Paper 533/2. Personal Social Services Research Unit (PSSRU), University of Kent, Canterbury.

—— & —— (1989) The cost-effectiveness of community care for former long-stay psychiatric hospital patients. Discussion Paper 628. PSSRU, University of Kent, Canterbury.

PRIEST, R. G. (1975) The homeless person and the psychiatric services: An Edinburgh survey. *British Journal of Psychiatry*, **128**, 128–136.

SHEPHERD, G. (1990) Case management. *Health Trends*, **22**, 59–62.

TIMMS, P. & FRY, A. (1989) Homelessness and mental illness. *Health Trends*, **21**, 70–71.

UK GOVERNMENT (1989*a*) *Caring for People. Community Care in the Next Decade and Beyond.* Cm 849. London: HMSO.

—— (1989*b*) *Working for Patients.* Cm 555. London: HMSO.

WOOFF, K. (ed.) (1989) Residential needs for severely disabled psychiatric patients: the case for hospital hostels. Key Workshop Papers. Manchester: Salford Health Authority. (Available from Mental Health Information Unit, Salford Health Authority, Pendleton House, Broughton Rd, Salford M6 6LQ).

YOUNG, R. (ed.) (1991) *Residential Needs for Severely Disabled Psychiatric Patients: The Case for Hospital Hostels.* London: HMSO.

Discussion: NIKOLAS MANOS

That services should be directed primarily towards the people who need them most is the starting point of Dr Shanks' paper. This emphasis on adequate services for people with persistent disability resulting from psychiatric illness is more than legitimate. It was also the main point that the US Commission on Mental Health made to the President in 1978: "An adequate, humane system of mental health care cannot exist until the special needs of Americans with long-term and severe mental disabilities are met, and until federal, state, and local governments share the responsibility for meeting this goal''.

Yet in the UK, as in the USA and, of course, elsewhere, there is a drift towards care of the 'worried well' in the community. In the case of these patients, Shanks says that primary care services, self-help, voluntary groups, and social services should accept the main responsibility for their treatment, but we also need to take into account the following realities.

Firstly, many people with other than psychotic disorders are also in great need of treatment.

Secondly, voluntary or self-help groups have proved efficient in some rehabilitation projects of the chronically mentally ill. Furthermore, it is debatable whether rehabilitation efforts, including housing, work, and socialisation, primarily need professional specialists or dedicated, non-specialist volunteers.

Thirdly, although the goal of strengthening the primary care doctor's ability to detect and treat at least minor psychiatric illness is worthy, many difficulties hamper this process. It is unclear as yet which patients can benefit from treatment in the primary care setting: systematic research in this area is so far lacking, and comparative data are needed on treatment by the primary care doctor versus the psychiatrist. In addition, research on the effectiveness of each type of treatment for different categories of patients is critical (Hankin & Oktay, 1979). When psychiatric disorders are classified according to the type of therapeutic intervention needed, e.g. major psychiatric illness, psychological distress syndromes not requiring intervention, and psychological distress syndromes that require intervention (Goldberg, 1982), it seems that the primary care doctor may be effective only in the second category. Although UK authors stress the need for strengthening the family doctor's therapeutic role (Shepherd *et al*, 1966), the US view stresses the need to train non-psychiatric doctors in the detection, management, and referral of persons with mental health problems (Goldberg *et al*, 1978).

In fact, the more specialised the treatment modalities that are available, e.g. a variety of specific psychotherapies, the greater the need for referral to a specialist. The danger of a two-level system of care, with a strengthening of the private sector serving many of the affluent 'worried well' is apparent.

Therefore, community psychiatric services should keep the care of the severely mentally ill as their first priority, but should also serve persons with all other psychiatric disorders. The community mental health centre of the Second University Department of Psychiatry in Thessaloníki, Greece, has implemented this type of broad synthetic model within the Greek National Health System for the past ten years.

Dr Shanks cites three studies which evaluated the cost-benefit advantage of placing patients in the community, in comparison with hospital-based care. The results are consistent with those from analogous studies (Smith & Hart, 1975; Murphy & Datel, 1976; Häfner & an der Heiden, 1989) in other countries, in that the community placement proves superior both in terms of cost and benefit, but only for less disabled patients. The cost in the community is higher for severely disabled patients, while for a small number neither system of care is effective in preventing chronicity (Smith & Hart, 1975).

In addition to hospital hostels as an alternative system of care, there are analogous systems such as the halfway house and the community residence, the evolution of which has been closely followed in the USA (Piasecki & Leary, 1980). An excellent description of a model halfway house run by two social workers led to the proposal that the money from deinstitutionalisation should be directed primarily to the establishment of halfway houses (Golomb & Kocsis, 1988). Yet cost is primarily related to the number of in-house services offered, i.e. the quality of the facility's functioning (Piasecki & Leary, 1980). For the evaluation of any kind of a community setting, however, "A judgment about any cost figure must be held in abeyance until one takes a closer look at the kind and quality of care. Programmes of active treatment will be far more expensive than custodial care" (Rubin, 1982).

The contribution of the clubhouse model in the provision of day care and sheltered work has been quite properly emphasised. The pioneering work at Fountain House (Beard *et al*, 1963) has emphasised the importance of the explicit recognition of mentally ill people as a resource, not merely as recipients of care. Research on Fountain House has already shown lower readmission rates, doubled length of stay in the community, and 40% fewer days in hospital for its residents, compared with controls (Beard *et al*, 1978). Newer clubhouses, such as the Open Door in Savannah, Georgia, have described ingenious rehabilitative work programmes, with former patients moving ahead through alternating cycles of progression, regression, and maintenance, each lasting four to five months, until they become able to hold independent jobs (Turkat, 1982). Other models of community residence and work, e.g. the work-orientated 'lodges' (from three to ten long-term patients living under the supervision of a counsellor and supporting themselves through group-work contracts [Beard *et al*, 1978]), have a similar philosophy.

Dr Shanks' emphasis on the importance of development in the area of management is certainly right. Every mental health agency needs a management information system (MIS), which is a mechanism for turning data into information to provide support for the manager, who must turn this information into decisions and plans (Paton & D'Huyvetter, 1980). In this context, 'manager' refers not only to executives and supervisors: any person charged with clinical, personnel, or organisational responsibility is a manager. Effective general management and case management should not only result in increased uptake of community resources, but also ensure high-quality continuity of care, which also depends on high-quality information. The four basic ingredients of continuity of care: client movement or lack of movement as a response to treatment needs, verbal and written communication among care-givers, stability of the client/care-giver relationship, and efforts to retrieve clients who appear to be prematurely dropping out of treatment (Ban, 1972), all rely on good case management.

The philosophy of the UK Griffiths Report is consistent with the proposal of Carter & Newman (1976) that a client-orientated system of mental health service delivery and programme management should be guided by two principles: that a local health programme is responsive to the demands placed on it by the community, and that it is accountable for what happens to its clients.

In agreement with Dr Shanks' stress on ''the need to specify and monitor the quality of our services as well as their volume'', there are many models for evaluating mental health treatment: organisational, care-process, consumer evaluation, efficacy, and community impact (Lebow, 1982). Optimal evaluation should include data relevant to each of the five models. It is always necessary to keep in mind that outcome is a change in a client's functioning concurrent with treatment, while effectiveness is a treatment-caused change in functioning (Fishman, 1981). Well-designed, multifactorial, controlled studies of cost-effectiveness are needed to evaluate the quality of our services.

It seems that in the UK, the USA, and most other countries, the dual system – institution and community services – will have to continue (Bachrach, 1983), with further improvements in both. A variety of highly successful programmes have enhanced the lives of some chronic psychiatric patients in most countries, albeit in varying degree. Yet, as Bachrach states, these are still too few in number to support the large population of patients who need care, and are too scattered to be of nationwide impact. Furthermore, professional staff and administrators are often either unaware of the relevant data concerning these successful models, or, when presented with the data, might discount or misuse them (Cook & Shadish, 1981). Surely, we can do better in the future.

References

BACHRACH, L. L. (1983) Evaluating the consequences of deinstitutionalisation. *Hospital and Community Psychiatry*, **34**, 105.
BAN, R. D. (1972) *A Method for Measuring Continuity of Care in a Community Mental Health Center*. US Department of Health and Human Services. NIMH Series C, no. 4. NIMH. 5600 Fishers Lane, Rockville, MD.
BEARD, J. H., SCHMIDT, J. R. & SMITH, M. M. (1963) The use of transitional employment in the rehabilitation of the psychiatric patient. *Journal of Nervous and Mental Disease*, **36**, 507–514.
BEARD, J. M., MALAMUD, T. J. & ROSSMAN, E. (1978) Psychiatric rehabilitation and long-term rehospitalisation rates; the findings of two research studies. *Schizophrenia Bulletin*, **4**, 622–635.

CARTER, D. E. & NEWMAN, F. L. (1976) *A Client-Oriented System of Mental Health Service Delivery and Progam Management. A Workbook and Guide.* Mental Health Service System Reports. Series FN, no. 4. US Department of Health and Human Services. NIMH. 5600 Fishers Lane, Rockville, MD.

COMMISSION ON MENTAL HEALTH (1978) *Report to the President from the President's Commission on Mental Health.* Washington, DC: US Government Printing Office.

COOK, T. & SHADISH, W. (1981) Meta-evaluation: an evaluation of the CMHC congressionally mandated evaluation system. In *Innovative Approaches to Mental Health Evaluation* (eds G. Stahler & W. Tash). New York: Academic Press.

FISHMAN, D. B. (1981) *A Cost-Effectiveness Methodology for Community Mental Health Centers: Development and Pilot Test.* Mental Health Service System Reports. Series FN, No. 3. US Department of Health and Human Services. NIMH. 5600 Fishers Lane, Rockville, MD.

GOLDBERG, D. P. (1982) The concept of a psychiatric 'case' in general practice. *Social Psychiatry*, **17**, 61–65.

——, BABIGIAN, H. M., LOCKE, B. Z., *et al* (1978) Role of nonpsychiatrist physicians in the delivery of mental health services. Implications from three studies. *Public Health Reports*, **93**, 240–245.

GOLOMB, S. K. & KOCSIS, A. (1988) *The Halfway House: On the road to Independence.* New York: Bruner/Mazel.

HÄFNER, H. & AN DER HEIDEN, W. (1989) Effectiveness and cost of community care for schizophrenic patients. *Hospital and Community Psychiatry*, **40**, 59–63.

HANKIN, J. & OKTAY, J. S. (1979) *Mental Disorder and Primary Medical Care: An Analytical Review of the Literature.* NIMH Series D, no. 5, US Department of Health and Human Services. NIMH. 5600 Fishers Lane, Rockville, MD.

LEBOW, J. (1982) Models for evaluating services at community mental health centers. *Hospital and Community Psychiatry*, **33**, 1010–1014.

MURPHY, J. G. & DATEL, W. E. (1976) A cost-benefit analysis of community versus institutional living. *Hospital and Community Psychiatry*, **27**, 165–170.

PATON, J. A. & D'HUYVETTER, P. K. (1980) *Automated Management Information Systems for Mental Health Agencies: A Planning and Acquisition Guide.* Mental Health Service System Reports. Series FN, no. 1. US Department of Health and Human Services. NIMH. 5600 Fishers Lane, Rockville, MD.

PIASECKI, J. R. & LEARY, J. E. (1980) *Halfway Houses and Long-term Community Residences for the Mentally Ill.* Mental Health Service System Reports. Series CN, no. 1. US Department of Health and Social Services. NIMH. 5600 Fishers Lane, Rockville, MD.

RUBIN, J. (1982) Cost measurement and cost data in mental health settings. *Hospital and Community Psychiatry*, **33**, 751–754.

SHEPHERD, M., COOPER, B., BROWN, A. C., *et al* (1966) *Psychiatric Illness in General Practice.* Oxford: Oxford University Press.

TURKAT, D. (1982) Psychosocial rehabilitation: a process evaluation. *Hospital and Community Psychiatry*, **33**, 848–850.

SMITH, W. G. & HART, D. W. (1975) Community mental health: a noble failure? *Hospital and Community Psychiatry*, **26**, 581–583.

5 Effectiveness of the wider social network in community care of the mentally ill

JORIS CASSELMAN

Before specialised institutions existed, care for the mentally ill was in fact community care; the foster-family care in Geel (Belgium), which started in the 13th century, has often been described as 'the birthplace' of such care (Srole, 1975; Roosens, 1977). However, even in Roman times, home care existed, as can be seen in a rescript of the Emperor Marcus Aurelius at the end of the 2nd century: an insane man who killed his mother was ordered to be kept at home, with paid guardians to care for his health and belongings (Spruit, 1976).

However, in most European countries, the latest movement of deinstitutionalisation has mainly been inspired by economic constraints. As a result of several waves of this process, a diverse delivery system of community services has been developed throughout many catchment areas. The phrase 'the wider social network in community care' was chosen for this chapter in order to capture the whole *Gestalt* of alternatives to traditional mental hospitals within a given community – not only the specialised professional services, but also the non-professional services. A list of community-based support staff and systems should include: day-care centres, night-care centres, after-care clinics, community mental health centres, crisis intervention centres, sheltered work settings, rehabilitation centres, sheltered living settings, halfway houses, nursing homes, hostels, board and care houses, supervised apartments, foster family care homes, family doctors, self-help groups, voluntary groups, family members, and friends.

Very often, however, networks of both professional and non-professional support systems are poorly organised and inadequately coordinated and integrated within a given community. This is one reason that many people remain doubtful about the effectiveness of these networks. Effectiveness in health planning has been defined by the WHO as "the degree to which a plan, a programme, or a project has achieved its purpose within the limits set for reaching its objective" (WHO, 1978).

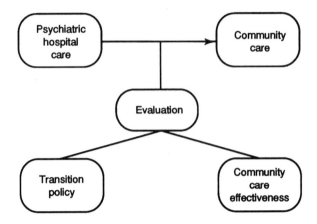

Fig. 5.1. Evaluation of transition policy and community care effectiveness in the transition from psychiatric hospital care to community care

This paper will consider only those mentally ill who have stayed for a long time or repeatedly in a traditional psychiatric hospital, or who would have done so in the past. It will first elaborate a formulation of the general problem, and then consider the current position in various European countries.

The general problem

The evaluation of the transition from psychiatric hospital care to community care for the mentally ill is a very complex issue; most frequently, it is limited to the study of national and regional statistics of psychiatric hospital populations. In a limited number of catchment areas, however, case-register data are available which reveal the career patterns over time of psychiatric patients through the various agencies (Wing, 1981; ten Horn *et al*, 1986). Evaluation of the effectiveness of the community care offered to the mentally ill, once discharged from the psychiatric hospital, is a rather neglected field (Fig. 5.1).

To consider the general problem more deeply, we shall next relate evaluation of the effectiveness of community care to a broader perspective of programme evaluation (Beenackers, 1986).

Effectiveness evaluation and programme evaluation

Mental health care evaluation research was originally limited to the evaluation of effects, but the broader concept of programme evaluation now

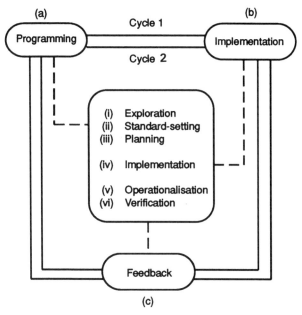

Fig. 5.2. Programme evaluation: three agencies and six phases

used includes a whole range, from the evaluation of a policy to that of a particular treatment. Moreover, a basic model has been conceptualised that is useful for all types of evaluation.

Adequate programme evaluation consists of a cyclic, feedback process, with one cycle including, successively, programming, implementation, and feedback. After a given activity has been programmed and implemented, its actual result is then compared with the intended result. Each cycle can be divided into six phases: exploration, standard-setting, and planning – all the responsibility of a programming or policy-making agency – the implementation phase, executed by an appropriate agency; and, finally, operationalisation and verification, both of which are realised by a feedback agency (Fig. 5.2). If necessary, the activity is reprogrammed and implemented once (or several times) more, and its result again (and again) compared with the intended result.

Evaluation of the effectiveness of community care

Psychiatric hospital staff are under growing pressure to make referrals to community services which have very different structures and offer different intensities of help to patients. The key question here is: what type of patient functions best in what type of community setting? This brings in the difficult issue of an operational definition of a patient's level of functioning.

Appropriate assessments of the characteristics of both patients and community settings are necessary. Moreover, the predictive value has to be evaluated of particular characteristics of patients in relation to successful functioning in one or another community setting (Braff & Lefkowitz, 1979).

The degree of ability to maintain a minimal level of psychosocial functioning in a particular community cannot be sufficiently predicted by traditional variables such as diagnosis and length of stay in hospital. Measurements have to be made directly in terms of levels of performance of social roles (Wing, 1981).

General critique

Every review of the research literature on the effectiveness of the community care of the mentally ill reaches similar conclusions: the literature is extensive, but characterised by a striking lack of methodological rigour and consistency. Only a limited number of studies have been prospective and have used control groups in an appropriate way. The reliable studies that do exist are not entirely comparable, a fact which is due to the differences in patient samples, measures of outcome, treatment settings, and lengths of follow-up. Frequently, the only outcome measure studied has been readmission to hospital: the rationale that these rates can easily be defined and that they have an economic justification does not excuse the fact that they are too narrow measures (Braff & Lefkowitz, 1979).

Outcome variables

While the findings on readmission rates are somewhat conflicting, some community programmes do help discharged patients to remain in the community. However, few studies take into account ex-patients' well-being, interpersonal functioning, and degree of instrumental role performance. In many studies, success in terms of avoiding admission automatically presumes individual well-being. If levels of functioning are evaluated, however, the most commonly used variables are symptomatology, social functioning, and employment.

An excellent review of the research literature (Braff & Lefkowitz, 1979) found only six well-designed studies which had used control groups, and in which at least three of the four variables (admission, symptomatology, social functioning, and employment) were found to be positive. The community care programmes studied varied greatly. Two combined drug treatment and therapy programmes for schizophrenics (Pasamanick *et al*, 1967; Hogarty *et al*, 1974), while the others consisted of aftercare in community mental health centres (Saenger, 1970), day hospitals (Herz *et al*, 1971), landlord-supervised apartments for schizophrenics (Chien & Cole, 1973), and training in community living (Test & Stein, 1977). The least frequently used were variables such as self-concept, perception of the sick role, and family pressure. Taking into consideration these variables, we may note that some community programmes do seem to be real alternatives to traditional mental hospital care. Community care is also, in general, less expensive, except for the most severely disabled (Murpay & Datel, 1976; Golomb & Kocsis, 1988; Häfner & an der Heiden, 1989).

Network of services in community care

The types of community care evaluated in effectiveness studies are very different, but one of the limitations of this work is that often only one community service or only one particular programme is studied. In reality, however, many discharged psychiatric patients seem to stay in the community because of a unique combination of different support persons and support systems, but this means that 'community support networks' are much more difficult to evaluate in an adequate way (Cutler *et al*, 1987).

As reviews of studies on social networks and psychosocial integration have shown, the concept of social network is useful in examining both functional and dysfunctional influences in the social reintegration of the mentally ill (Froland *et al*, 1979; Mitchell & Trickett, 1980; Häfner & Welz, 1988). An example of the combination of several services in the same programme, as an alternative to in-patient care, is the day-hospital-inn programme developed by the Massachusetts Mental Health Center in Boston (Goudeman *et al*, 1985; Gersons & Perguin, 1987). The 'training in community living' (TCL) model is an example of an intensive training of the mentally ill to live in the community, instead of being admitted to a traditional psychiatric hospital (Stein & Test, 1985; Hoult, 1986).

The situation in Europe

Recent reviews of the very complex situation of mental health policy, implementation, and evaluation in Europe are in agreement about several important issues (Freeman *et al*, 1985; WHO, 1988; Groot, 1989; De Haen, 1989). Firstly, in almost all countries, mental health care is in the process of reorientation and reorganisation. The main themes are: prevention of unnecessary admissions, shortening the length of residential stay, ensuring continuity of care, differentiation of care, decentralisation of organisations, and integration of mental health care into general health care and social welfare. Many of these options fit the more general policy of transition from traditional psychiatric hospital care to community care.

However, there is also a consensus with regard to the generally slow implementation and obviously limited availability of evaluation data. Overall, actual implementation is slower than is generally thought, but its intensity and tempo are still very different from one country to another.

In the field of evaluation of mental health care, much more information is available on general policy than on the effectiveness of community care (Sand & Baro, 1981; Freeman *et al*, 1985; WHO, 1988; De Haen, 1989; Groot, 1989). For policy evaluation, existing official statistics are most frequently used; sometimes international inquiries, visits, or expert meetings provide additional information and, exceptionally, data from psychiatric case registers are available (Sand & Baro, 1981; ten Horn, 1981; Giel *et al*, 1984; Freeman *et al*, 1985; ten Horn *et al*, 1986; WHO, 1987, 1988; De Haen, 1989; Groot, 1989).

Psychiatric case registers provide valuable material that can help to evaluate the use of complementary community services in particular geographical areas, and to compare one area with another in the same country or in other countries (Giel & ten Horn, 1984; ten Horn *et al*, 1986; WHO, 1987). In a study in West Germany, the findings of an existing psychiatric case register were combined with additional research data in order to evaluate the effectiveness of components of the community care for schizophrenics (Häfner & an der Heiden, 1986). A total of 18 months' detailed registration of contacts with services was divided into a first period of 12 months and a second period of six months. The effect was studied of care variables on symptoms during the first period, while the frequency and length of readmission during the second period was also investigated. The main variables were operationalised as follows: (a) course of the illness before the observation period, by considering all former hospital treatments; (b) psychopathology, by means of the Present State Examination's subscores for BSO (behaviour, speech, and other disorders); and (c) out-patient care, by calculating the number of monthly contacts during the observation period spent outside hospital. Significant correlations were found, on the one hand, between the intensity of out-patient treatment during the first period and the decline of psychopathological disturbances, and, on the other hand, the frequency of readmission during the second period. Generally speaking, in many countries in Europe, a general evaluative picture of the transition policy can be drawn, but little research has been undertaken on the effectiveness of community care for the mentally ill.

This is even the case for a country such as Italy with an exceptionally abrupt mental health law reform in 1978, generating much research interest both within and outside the country (Misiti, 1981; Giel & ten Horn, 1984; Freeman *et al*, 1985; Vanistendael, 1985; WHO, 1987; Crepet, 1988; WHO, 1988; Van der Poel & Haafkens, 1989). In a review of the valuation research (Crepet, 1988), it was clearly stated that little is known about the fate of those discharged from the traditional psychiatric hospitals. On the general policy level, the available data demonstrate that the impact of the reform is very different from one area to another.

In some parts of Italy, the community services seem to provide a high quality of care, but in other parts, because of the lack of appropriate community services, the attitudes of the general public and family members of the mentally ill, and the low degree of interest of politicians and local administrators, widespread use is made of both psychiatric and non-psychiatric residential settings. Crepet's review of evaluation research in Italy (1988) mentions only the following data on the discharged chronically mentally ill. In the Venice area, of those discharged, 86% were still alive two years later and 60% of these lived in private houses, 34% were in non-psychiatric institutions, 13% had jobs, and 54% were receiving the attention of psychiatric or social services. The Piedmont region, however, showed a different picture: 43% of those discharged were living in psychiatric hospital wards converted into apartments, 40% were living in community residences, and 12% were homeless. Crepet cites not even one well-designed study with a control group, investigating the effectiveness of community care.

Evaluation of the effectiveness of community care for the mentally ill is also a neglected research field in other parts of Europe. This is especially the case if one looks for well-designed studies with control groups, adequate outcome variables, and an orientation towards the network of community services (Jones, 1985; Hyde *et al*, 1987; Tansella & Williams, 1987; Tansella *et al*, 1987; Northeast Thames Regional Health Authority, 1988; Mosher & Burti, 1989).

The selection of pilot study regions which have long-standing experience with psychiatric case registers and are willing to combine this basic material with additional research seems to be one of the possible research pathways that should be followed.

Conclusion

The limited objective of this paper was to elaborate a general problem formulation for the evaluation of the effectiveness of the wider social network in community care of the mentally ill. One possible recommendation is to take as a frame of reference a basic programme-evaluation model that is useful for all types of evaluation, e.g. general policy, effectiveness. The research literature on the effectiveness of community care of the mentally ill is characterised by a striking lack of methodological rigour and uniformity. Difficult areas are the prospective perspective, control groups, outcome variables, and the network of community services.

Since these limitations can be observed in Europe generally, pilot study regions having a long-standing experience with psychiatric case registers should be motivated to combine these data with additional research findings,

64   *Casselman*

enabling the evaluation of the effectiveness of community care to be put
on a sounder footing.

References

BEENACKERS, A. A. J. M. (1986) *Project-evaluatie in de geestelijke gezondheidszorg.* Delft: Eburon.
BRAFF, J. & LEFKOWITZ, M. M. (1979) Community mental health treatment: what works for
  whom?, *Psychiatric Quarterly*, **51**, 119–134.
CHIEN, C. & COLE, J. (1973) Landlord supervised cooperative apartments: a new modality
  for community-based treatment. *American Journal of Psychiatry*, **130**, 156–159.
CREPET, P. (1988) The Italian mental health reform nine years on. *Acta Psychiatrica Scandinavica*,
  938, 1–9.
CUTLER, D. L., TATUM, E. & SHORE, J. H. (1987) A comparison of schizophrenic patients
  in different community support treatment approaches. *Community Mental Health Journal*, **23**,
  103–113.
DE HAEN, F. (ed.) (1989) *De GGZ in enkele Europese landen (België, Frankrijk, Engeland, Wales,
  Denemarken en Zwitserland).* Utrecht: Nationaal Ziekenhuisinstituut.
FREEMAN, H. L., FRYERS, T. & HENDERSON, J. A. (1985) *Mental Health Services in Europe: 10
  Years on.* Copenhagen: WHO Regional Office for Europe.
FROLAND, C., BRODSKY, G., OLSON, M., *et al* (1979) Social support and social adjustment:
  implications for mental health professionals. *Community Mental Health Journal*, **15**, 82–93.
GERSONS, B. P. R. & PERQUIN, L. N. M. (1987) Het dagziekenhuis-herbergmodel: alternatief
  voor 24-uurs psychiatrische opname. *Tijdschrift voor Psychiatrie*, **29**, 621–637.
GIEL, R. & TEN HORN, G. H. M. M. (1984) Triëst in 1984. *Maandblad Geertelijhe Volksgezondheid*,
  39, 946–952.
GOLOMB, S. L. & KOCSIS, A. (1988) *The Half-way House: On the Road to Independence.* New York:
  Brunner/Mazel.
GOUDEMAN, J. E., DICKEY, B., EVANS, A., *et al* (1985) Four-years' assessment of a day-
  hospital-inn program as an alternative to in-patient hospitalization. *American Journal of Psychiatry*,
  142(11), 1330–1333.
GROOT, L. (1989) *Evaluatie van de psychiatrische ziekenhuisprogrammatie.* Brussels: Ministerie
  Volksgezondheid.
HÄFNER, H. & AN DER HEIDEN, W. (1986) The Mannheim case register: the long-stay
  population. In *Psychiatric Case Registers in Public Health* (eds G. H. M. M. ten Horn, R. Giel,
  W. H. Gulbinat, *et al*), pp. 28–38. Amsterdam, New York: Elsevier.
—— & —— (1989) Effectiveness and cost of community care for schizophrenic patients.
  Hospital and Community Psychiatry, **40**, 59–63.
—— & WELZ, R. (1988) Social networks and mental disorder (with special reference to the
  elderly). In *Health and Behaviour: Selected Perspectives* (eds D. Hamburg & N. Sartorius),
  pp. 150–161. Cambridge: Cambridge University Press.
HERZ, M., ENDICOTT, J., SPITZER, R., *et al* (1971) Day versus in-patient hospitalization: a
  controlled study. *American Journal of Psychiatry*, **127**, 1371–1381.
HOGARTY, G., GOLDBERG, S., SCHOOLER, N., *et al* (1974) Drug and sociotherapy in the
  aftercare of schizophrenic patients. II: Two-year relapse rates. *Archives of General Psychiatry*,
  31, 603–608.
HOULT, J. (1986) Community care of the mentally ill. *British Journal of Psychiatry*, **149**, 137–144.
HYDE, C., BRIDGES, K., GOLDBERG, D., *et al* (1987) The evaluation of a hostel ward: a
  controlled study using modified cost-benefit analysis. *British Journal of Psychiatry*, **151**, 805–812.
JONES, K. (1985) *After hospital: a study of long-term psychiatric patients in York.* York:
  University of York and York Health Authority.
MISITI, R. (1981) The state of psychiatric care one year after the coming into effect of Law
  180. In *Evaluation and Mental Health Care* (eds E. A. Sand & F. Baro), pp. 129–148.
  Luxembourg: Commission of the European Countries.

MITCHELL, R. E. & TRICKETT, E. J. (1980) Task force report: social networks as mediators of social support. *Community Mental Health Journal*, **16**, 27–44.

MOSHER, L. R. & BURTI, L. (1989) *Community Mental Health: Principles and Practice*. New York: Norton.

MURPAY, J. G. & DATEL, W. E. (1976) A cost-benefit analysis of community versus institutional living. *Hospital and Community Psychiatry*, **27**, 165–170.

NORTH EAST THAMES REGIONAL HEALTH AUTHORITY (1988) *TAPS. Team for the Assessment of Psychiatric Services. Preliminary Report on Baseline Data from Friern and Claybury Hospitals*. London: NETRHA.

PASAMANICK, B., SCARPITTI, F. & DINITZ, S. (1967) *Schizophrenics in the Community*. New York: Appleton-Century-Crofts.

ROOSENS, E. (1977) *Geel, een unicum in de psychiatrie*. Antwerp: De Nederlandsche Boekhandel.

SAENGER, G. (1970) Patterns of change among treated and untreated patients seen in psychiatric community mental health clinics. *Journal of Nervous and Mental Disease*, **150**, 37–50.

SAND, E. A. & BARO, F. (eds) (1981) *Evaluation and Mental Health Care*. Third European Seminar on Health Policy. Luxembourg: Commission of the European Communities.

SPRUIT, J. E. (1976) Opvattingen van Marcus Aurelius omtrent de strafrechterlijke aansprakelijkheid van en voor geestelijk gestoorden. In *Recht, macht en manipulatie* (eds C. Kelk, *et al*), pp. 480–510. Utrecht: Spectrum, Aula.

SROLE, L., (1975) *The Geel family care research project*. Geel: International Symposium on Family Care for the Mentally Ill.

STEIN, L. I. & TEST, M. A. (eds) (1985) *The Training in Community Living Model: A Decade of Experience*. San Francisco: Jossey-Bass.

TANSELLA, M., DE SALVIA, D. & WILLIAMS, P. (1987) The Italian psychiatric reform: some quantative evidence. *Social Psychiatry*, **22**, 37–48.

—— & WILLIAMS, P. (1987) The Italian experience and its implications. *Psychological Medicine*, **17**, 283–289.

TEN HORN, G. H. M. M. (1981) The use of a mental health case register for the evaluation of mental health policy. In *Evaluation and Mental Health Care* (eds E. A. Sand & F. Baro), pp. 149–163. Luxembourg: Commission of the European Communities.

——, GIEL, R., GULBINAT, W. H., *et al* (eds) (1986) *Psychiatric Case Registers in Public Health*. Amsterdam: Elsevier.

TEST, M. & STEIN, L. (1977) A community approach to the chronically disabled patient. *Policy*, **8**, 8–16.

VAN DER POEL, E. & HAAFKENS, J. (1989) Italia quo vadis? *Perspectief*, **7**, 3–20.

VANISTENDAEL, C. (1985) Prevention of admission and continuity of care. *Theoretical Medicine*, **6**, 93–113.

WHO (1978) *Glossary of Health Care Terminology* (J. Hogarth). Copenhagen: WHO Regional Office for Europe.

—— (1987) *Mental Health Services in Pilot Study Areas*. Report on a European study. Copenhagen: WHO, Regional Office for Europe.

—— (1988) *Mental Health Services in Southern Countries of the European Region*. Copenhagen: WHO.

WING, J. K. (1981) Evaluation of mental health services: principles and methods of measurement. In *Evaluation and Mental Health Care* (eds E. A. Sand & F. Baro), pp. 21–34. Third European Seminar on Health Policy. Luxembourg: Commission of the European Communities.

Discussion: ROGER AMIEL

This paper focuses on those severely mentally ill patients who have stayed for a prolonged time, and those who are detained repeatedly, in a traditional psychiatric hospital. Should we consider further the kinds of patients concerned, and also the question of what is considered to be a traditional psychiatric hospital?

To narrow the discussion, we could assume that such severely ill patients are mainly psychotic and schizophrenic: their mental disorders would have begun early in their lives, at about the age of 20, and have lasted for some 20 to 30 years. Thus, their hospital stay began 20–30 years ago, at a time when the 'traditional' psychiatric hospital was as yet generally an institution without out-patient facilities or any network of community care. Yet no active psychiatric hospital could adequately or competently care for and treat such patients today without these extramural services.

However, there are other types of psychiatric patients whose condition may also be considered severe: the majority of these – as it did 20–30 years ago – consists of the elderly who suffer from dementia. They are admitted much later in their lives than are the schizophrenics, and their treatment is more or less standardised in long-term, specialised care centres, where there are clean and decent living conditions. They need not be discussed further here. Two other types of patients use the modern psychiatric hospital during their acute phases: those with serious neurotic disorders, who usually come to seek help for a few days, and some manic–depressives, who more and more often prefer to be treated in the psychiatric ward of a general hospital for a few weeks. They also will not be discussed in detail here.

Focusing mainly on the severely ill schizophrenic patients, we find that most have left the hospital setting since their illness began. Darcourt *et al* (1989) in a retrospective study over 10 years of 383 schizophrenic patients, notes that the average length of their hospital stay was about 20 months in total, or an average of two months per year. Where were they and how were they followed-up when not in hospital during these 10 years? They were to be found in that wide range of out-care centres and community services of which Dr Casselman gives a long list – about one-quarter were in intensive psychotherapy in after-care homes, or at day hospitals; the rest were in diverse ambulatory settings (receiving an average of from 7 to 8 consultations per year). Of the 383 patients (with an average age of a little less than 40), 6% (24) had died (9 by suicide): 51 patients were lost to follow-up and their condition unknown. Of the remaining 308 patients, only one was no longer diagnosed as schizophrenic; thus, after 10 years, only one patient was classified as completely cured.

How can we know if these extramural facilities are well used and efficient? How can we measure the effectiveness of these alternative social and community psychiatric centres, where there are few doctors, medication is optional, and lay members of the community may be offering emotional help to patients?

Dr Casselman was concerned with the *Gestalt* formed by the different components of the social network for the mentally ill in a given community. A gestalt figure or structure is characterised by unity, integration, wholeness, and coherence; an analysis of it begins with the whole and proceeds through a continuum to the parts. Gestalt psychology emphasises inherent potential, values the external forces, and identifies the distortions between alienated parts, thus helping to re-establish the conditions under which individuals can best use their own problem-solving and communication skills. In this manner, the gestalt of a psychiatric system can be perceived only as a dynamic whole, and only its components can be described or analysed in detail. Looking for the effectiveness of such a gestalt of community-based support of people and systems is a way to understand how its institutions can work in harmony and symbiosis.

But to avoid patients being lost from follow-up, we must maintain their 'transfer' (in the psychoanalytical sense), not to a single therapist, but more to a team, and even better to a range of institutions, integrated into a network (gestalt) upon which the patients can rely. In France, such a community network is called a *secteur*, but those who see in the word only the idea of a geographical catchment area are wrong. The *secteur* is in fact a team which has a single director and the ability to coordinate diverse and flexible methods for the follow-up mainly of the young psychotics who reside specifically within a given community, which is not necessarily geographically limited. Such communities can also consist of people belonging to a single profession (e.g. farm workers, teachers). This adds the notion of solidarity to community care.

Is it possible to evaluate the effectiveness of the care and maintenance of this type of patient within a *secteur*? I have myself launched three such pilot enterprises, which have normally included an evaluation system of the work carried out. Were the results of these studies significant? They were, in terms of understanding what happens in each separate institution – how each functions in terms of input and output. This is descriptive epidemiology: a minimum of it is necessary for budget reasons. If we want to obtain a wider perception of the overall function of the network by following up the patients, it is possible to limit the number of variables and parameters to only three or four, e.g. diagnosis, age, length of stay, and type of medication. This is analytical epidemiology in a prospective sense, which allows us to follow the evolution of a small group of patients, fewer than 50, but not to compare them with those of another *secteur*. Nor can it answer questions such as – what is the correlation between particular interventions and the likelihood of returning to employment?

I agree therefore with Dr Casselman's relative pessimism when he reviews the literature about the effectiveness of comprehensive psychiatric services. When there were only traditional psychiatric hospitals, it was easier to gather statistics on length of hospital stay or the number of relapses. Today this is almost impossible, if we want to follow the complete progress of a very large number of patients. How can we calculate, for instance, the impact of the number of telephone calls from nurses to the patients living in their own homes?

What is more feasible is to outline the gestalt of the sectorial services available to a given group of people, and to examine how the members of the professional teams of the different institutions communicate and cooperate with each other. The objective is essentially to improve the effectiveness of the different components making up a community care and treatment system. But its results cannot be compared with those of other *secteurs* because the patients, staff, numbers of patients, degree of community acceptance, etc. are simply not comparable.

We should also be aware of the current limitations in the effectiveness of both psychotherapy and psychopharmacology. Although most psychotic people are no longer in hospitals, they are still conspicuously in need of further and continued treatment. As the demand for custodial care lessens, psychiatry further emphasises the social context of its responsibilities, and puts the accent on rehabilitation which is delivered within community-based services, involving a gestalt of small psychiatric centres. Instead of starting our studies only from the base, i.e. from the patient, we should also examine how the whole gestalt of a *secteur* mobilises its different personnel and institutions, in order to see how they cope with both chronically handicapped and acutely ill patients.

Reference

DARCOURT *et al* (1989) Evolution des psychoses. Résultats d'une enquite sur 383 cas suivis pendant 10 ans. *Annales Medico-Psychologiques*, **147**, 15–32.

6 Evaluation of change in the system of mental health care

DURK WIERSMA and ROBERT GIEL

Since the 1960s, the number of mental hospital beds per 1000 of the population has been decreasing in European countries, but this change seems to have had a limited effect on numbers of personnel and size of budgets (WHO, 1971, 1980, 1986; EEC, 1981; Freeman *et al*, 1985; Mangen, 1985). Although the general decline continued into the 1980s, there are signs that further reductions would be difficult (Carling *et al*, 1987; Ford *et al*, 1987; Häfner, 1987; Dorwart, 1988).

Nevertheless, mental health care policy in most countries is still focusing on less use of hospitals, but more community care and sheltered accommodation outside hospital. However, the use of ambulatory and domiciliary care instead of institutional mental hospital care affects quite different patient populations: long-stay patients from 'back wards' (requiring substitution at the end-point of the institution); chronic patients with frequent admissions of intermediate duration; acute, short-stay patients (substitution at the entry point); and specific patient populations in day hospitals, day centres, etc. It is evident that shorter stay in hospital, together with changes in discharge policy and the growth of rehabilitation, has altered the objectives and organisation of hospital care, although little is known about the magnitude and quality of these changes.

The WHO Pilot Areas Study (WHO, 1987) indicated that in the early 1980s, in most countries of Europe, a schizophrenic patient with an acute episode was nearly always admitted for at least a brief period of time and had hardly any out-patient contacts during the follow-up period of two years. Continuity of care was rare. The data showed very little evidence of community care, and one wonders whether the situation is much different today. Deinstitutionalisation has drawn attention to some serious drawbacks of institutional care, to the precarious civil rights of committed patients, and to some appropriate alternatives to the hospital. However, it is time to assess and evaluate the changes that have occurred in the mental health care systems of European countries.

Deinstitutionalisation in the 1980s: some models

The process of deinstitutionalisation has followed various pathways. Stein & Test (1980), for example, developed their 'Training in Community Living' model in Madison, Wisconsin (USA); this was later replicated by Hoult *et al* (1983) in Sydney (Australia), using mobile treatment teams, community nursing, and living-skills centres. In both cases, drastic changes in the system of care resulted, and these were thoroughly investigated, with positive outcomes. Important features were abolishing the central role of the mental hospital, and providing comprehensive and integrated mental health care in close collaboration with other medical (GP) and social services.

Another example of this kind of system can be found in Italy (e.g. Arezzo, Trieste, South Verona). Replacement of all hospital care by community care is the main objective (Tansella *et al*, 1987*a* and *b*; Mosher & Burti, 1989).

Another trend is that of splitting up the mental hospital into smaller units to be located in the more populated areas, with the aim of promoting rehabilitation in the community. Beds remain, but their use is much more specific to particular patient populations (e.g. therapeutic community, borderline patients, addiction unit). The hospital survives because of its new functions, while local circumstances determine the feasibility of community care and to what extent reinstitutionalisation in other forms (in hostels or sheltered homes) can be prevented. Much depends on the balanced mixture of hospital and community services, as is demonstrated by the systems of care in Worcestershire (UK) (Hall & Brockington, 1991), and in Melbourne (Australia) with its conglomerate of mental hospitals known as 'Psychopolis'.

Sometimes a hospital updates its public image by providing day treatment instead of full-time hospital care, or by offering hotel facilities. A good example is the hospital 'inn' model promoted by Gudeman *et al* (1983) in Boston (USA), or the partial hospitalisation programme of Herz *et al* (1972). In some countries, psychiatric units with services reaching out into the community are neglected. These examples show the multitude of solutions sought in various countries, or even within the same country. There is no 'gold standard' of community care.

Changes of what kind?

The changes to be observed depend on the perspective of the observer. Change can be defined in terms of the product (e.g. admissions, episodes of care, types of care), of the effect (e.g. number of disabled people, degree of resocialisation, relief from distress or burden), of cost (total amount of money, proportion of total health care costs, cost of hospital care versus ambulatory care), and of organisation (e.g. network of institutions, kind of personnel, level of training).

From the perspective of deinstitutionalisation, one must evaluate changes in the utilisation of mental hospital beds and in the provision of care in the community (cf. Dowell & Ciarlo, 1983). The latter is supposed to solve a number of problems associated with traditional care: overemphasis on residential treatment, insufficient emphasis on patients' social functioning and social situation, low level of training of mental health personnel, lack of cohesion of services, inadequate after-care, discontinuous care, neglect of the long-stay patient, etc.

Because of the manifold systems of care in various countries, it is difficult to evaluate these changes comparatively. For example, what is currently the content of in-patient care in various countries (McCready *et al*, 1985; Wolff *et al*, 1989)? Much depends on the facilities and the kind of personnel 'around the bed' as to whether admission use is good or bad. Quantity and quality of care are difficult to assess or compare, as are its therapeutic elements (Goldstein & Horgan, 1988). The same applies to community care (e.g. Kunze, 1985; Jones *et al*, 1986). Finally, the quality of life of both patients and their relatives have to be considered.

Most evaluation reports tell very little about the effects of a new programme on the total health care system in a country, thereby preventing its generalisation to others. Psychiatric epidemiology of the last 20 to 30 years (Hare & Wing, 1970; Strömgren *et al*, 1980; Williams *et al*, 1989) nevertheless shows that modest progress has occurred in evaluation research. However, evaluative evidence regarding the adequacy and effectiveness of change is scarce (Wing, 1982; Hyde *et al*, 1987), although there has been much improvement in the measurement and classification of psychopathological phenomena, as well as in that of social disability, social support, social network, etc.

Nevertheless, psychiatric case registers (ten Horn *et al*, 1986) and longitudinal (cross-cultural) research, sometimes in experimental designs (Fenton *et al*, 1979; Stein & Test, 1980; Cullberg & Stefansson, 1981; Häfner & Klug, 1982; Hoult *et al*, 1983; Munk-Jorgensen, 1985), have yielded a wealth of descriptive data, assisting the evaluation and planning of community mental health care.

In order to study change, some form of programme evaluation is necessary: this means establishing the value of a programme by comparing its effects with its objectives (Suchman, 1967; Guttentag & Struening, 1975; Struening & Guttentag, 1975; Coursey *et al*, 1977). In the context of deinstitutionalisation, providing community care as a substitute for hospital care is a logical alternative objective. Häfner & an der Heiden (1989) have described a set of criteria for such an evaluation: precise description of the intervention, a homogeneous patient population with respect to intervention and outcome, and clear definition of therapeutic goals. Unfortunately, many studies in this area are deficient in design, and lack random assignment of patients; however, it may become clear that the changes disappear after some time, since they were merely due to a 'Hawthorne effect'. In order to overcome such deficiencies and the lack of generalisability, it is necessary to follow a comprehensive approach, if change in the total care system is to be evaluated (cf. Sartorius & Harding, 1983).

In the Netherlands, we are in the process of studying the impact of substituting day-treatment and community care for traditional residential care (Wiersma *et al*, 1989).

Substitution of hospital beds: a controlled study in the Netherlands

The objective of this evaluation is to establish the effects of the 'substitution model' with the help of a clinical trial. The control condition comprises conventional 24-hour residential care in the mental hospital, including routine out-patient after-care. The experimental condition consists of a new form of day treatment provided by the mental hospital for its adult patients, interwoven with ambulatory and domiciliary care offered by the social psychiatric service together with the out-patient department of the hospital, treatment which aims to avoid full-time hospital admission and create more continuity of care. The experiment is characterised by random allotment of patients on admission.

Criteria for entrance into the study are that patients should be:

(a) accepted for 24-hour hospital care according to ordinary admission criteria, and coming from a circumscribed, mainly rural area in one of the northern Dutch provinces with 95 000 inhabitants;
(b) aged 18 years or more;
(c) not suffering from dementia (ICD–9: 290, 291.1 and 2), and not referred for psychiatric examination by a court.

Subsequent to the index-admission, each patient will be followed-up for two years. Interviews with the patients and their relatives take place on admission, at six weeks, at one year, and finally at two years. Our psychiatric case register monitors the utilisation of mental health services during follow-up.

The impact of the 'substitution approach' and its differential effects will be evaluated on the following five levels, each with its own specific instruments and methodology.

Patient level

In this level the focus is on patients' functioning over a period of two years, with assessment of their psychiatric condition according to DSM–III–R criteria (American Psychiatric Association, 1987) and the Present State

Examination (Wing *et al*, 1974). Intellectual and psychological impairments are measured (Wiersma, 1986; Tholen *et al*, 1988), as well as the extent and course of social disability. This latter measurement uses the Groningen Social Disabilities Schedule (Wiersma *et al*, 1988), which includes questions about the social network and social support (derived from the Self-Esteem and Social Support Schedule of Brown *et al*, 1986).

Family level

In this level, the focus is on the burden on the family (Grad & Sainsbury, 1968; Creer *et al*, 1982), in cases where the patient lives in a family or household. An instrument specially developed for this study is directed at measuring the strains experienced, and the objective and subjective burden on the partner or a close relative, including actual social support given (Kluiter, 1987). In addition, the partner's degree of satisfaction with the patient's treatment and supervision is measured.

Care level

Here all treatment and care given both inside and outside the mental hospital are recorded, including time spent with the patient, the number of face-to-face contacts with other professionals or the family, and presence in or absence from the unit (particularly during nights or weekends, because during such times many patients are on leave). All therapeutic activities are enumerated. For contacts with other facilities than the hospital or social psychiatric service, the psychiatric case register is the main source of information (Giel & ten Horn, 1982). This register, initiated in 1974 according to the principles of the Camberwell register (Wing & Hailey, 1972), has covered the province of Drenthe, which includes our catchment area, since 1986.

Institutional level

At this level, the new approach is likely to affect the structure and culture of the whole hospital, its out-patient department, and the social psychiatric service. The analysis of such intra- and interorganisational changes includes questions concerning:

(a) effects on wards;
(b) input of staff;
(c) (re)training of staff;
(d) 7×24 hours on-call service of the social psychiatric services;
(e) domiciliary visits by clinical workers;
(f) time spent on consultation and patient–staff meetings;

(g) effects on workload of the social psychiatric service;
(h) cost of day treatment for each institution.

Level of the regional mental health care system

The regional system is characterised by a relative abundance of mental health facilities (Giel & ten Horn, 1982). The network consists of two other mental hospitals, several psychiatric departments in general hospitals, in- and out-patient clinics for alcohol and drug dependence, sheltered homes, social services, general practitioners, etc.

Issues of evaluation

In various countries (the USA, Italy, Australia, the UK), alternatives to full-time hospital admission have been shown to be effective, at least for certain groups of patients (Stein & Test, 1980; Braun *et al*, 1981; Herz, 1982; Bennett & Morris, 1983; Hoult, 1986; Schene & Gersons, 1986; Rosie, 1987; Tansella *et al*, 1987; Creed *et al*, 1989b; Mosher & Burti, 1989). Their feasibility depends on a variety of local, regional, and national factors, such as the availability of forceful advocates of the 'alternative', a positive attitude on the part of mental health workers, political goodwill, and appropriate funding, to mention a few.

Partial hospital admission, however, has never become a successful alternative for the seriously mentally ill (Luber, 1979; DiBella *et al*, 1982; Steinhart & Bosch, 1983; Vaughan, 1985; McGrath & Tantam, 1987; Creed *et al*, 1989a; Tantam & McGrath, 1989). Important questions relevant to the subject of feasibility are as follows:

(a) In what way can the elements operative in the new forms of day treatment best be described?
(b) What is the difference from ordinary residential care and from more traditional day care?
(c) To what extent can the new approach be maintained, once its initial charisma has worn off?
(d) Is it adequate according to professional standards, as well as in the opinion of patients and their families?
(e) What kind of training is necessary for the mental health workers?

In the context of total health care, the new system means replacing one type of care with another, while retaining the original functions for the same or a comparable population of patients. In this case, mental hospital beds are being replaced by an equal number of places in a day-treatment setting, while retaining the functions of treatment and round-the-clock care for patients who would previously have been admitted. The new approach should not, however, attract new categories of patients who otherwise would never have been admitted. In our view, residential care should still be available during the period of evaluation, when it is unavoidable, while, for the time being, day treatment should not automatically result in budgetary cuts. The objective is to show how many and what types of patients can be maintained in the new treatment setting, in order to identify predictors of success.

'Prevention' refers in this instance to reduction or avoidance of chronicity and disablement. Can the alternative really prevent long stay in hospital or frequent readmission? Does it result in better integration of patients into society? The gains for the patient should not be outweighed by increased health costs for the relatives. Other medical costs, e.g. extra medication and visits to general health services, should also be taken into account.

The 'functional coherence' of mental health care is an important objective of managers or policymakers. It serves the aims of efficiency and effectiveness. It is fundamental to the principle of continuity of care for a population of mostly chronic patients, to whom after-care is frequently not easily available. Both the costs and benefits of the alternative approach should be compared, at each of the levels of evaluation mentioned above.

Accountability (van de Poel, 1986) implies taking into account both debits and credits in money or service, in order to decide on cost allocation. A cost-benefit analysis is to be preferred to other methods of economic evaluation (see, e.g. Glass & Goldberg, 1977; Dickey *et al*, 1986; Drummond *et al*, 1987; Schwefel *et al*, 1988). The results of the analysis at each level should be incorporated into the overall cost-benefit analysis of the alternative treatment.

Conclusions

Systems of mental health care do not change easily. Hospital beds are still at the heart of planning and funding, although formal policy seems to point in a different direction (cf. Griffith report on community care in the UK, 1988). There are several models of change, each of which should be evaluated against criteria of adequacy, efficiency, and effectiveness. The practice of in-patient care, and other forms should be carefully described, including qualitative and quantitative changes over time. The scope of evaluation should be wide and comprehensive, covering all aspects of mental health care in a region. Patterns of care should be studied, instead of individual elements (Sytema *et al*, 1989).

Concepts of community care, continuity of care, etc. have to be properly operationalised; evaluation should become part of a continuous programme of work, in which planning and evaluation go hand in hand. Data on contacts with psychiatric services, as well as on the type and amount of mental health care provided at the primary care level, need to be collected. Therefore, innovations in care should be precisely formulated, jointly with the development of methodologically sound research (Helgason, 1983; Holland, 1983). The mental hospital should have a say in the development and implementation of alternative care, so that the system can also be reformed from within.

The success of innovations depends on the local situation in the network of services, as well as on the commitment of research foundations and university departments that are interested in evaluative research (Mosher & Burti, 1989). Innovative projects are important in the rationalisation of existing patterns of care, in improving criteria for acceptance into or referral to a service, and in promoting the quality of care in terms of adequacy, efficiency, and effectiveness.

References

AMERICAN PSYCHIATRIC ASSOCIATION (1987) *Diagnostic and Statistical Manual of Mental Disorders* (3rd edn, revised) (DSM–III–R).

BENNETT, D. & MORRIS, I. (1983) Deinstitutionalisation in the United Kingdom. *International Journal of Mental Health*, **2**, 5–23.

BRAUN, P., KOCHANSKY, G., SHAPIRO, R., *et al* (1981) Overview. Deinstitutionalisation of psychiatric patients. A critical review of outcome studies. *American Journal of Psychiatry*, **138**, 736–749.

BROWN, G. W., ANDREWS, B., HARRIS, T., *et al* (1986) Social support, self-esteem and depression. *Psychological Medicine*, **16**, 813–831.

CARLING, P. J., MILLER, S., DANIELS, L. V., *et al* (1987) A state mental health system with no state hospital: the Vermont feasibility study. *Hospital and Community Psychiatry*, **38**, 617–624.

COURSEY, R. D., SPECTER, G. A., MURRELL, S. A., *et al* (eds) (1977) *Program Evaluation for Mental Health: Methods, Strategies, and Participants*. New York: Grune & Stratton.

CREED, F., BLACK, D. & ANTHONY, P. (1989*a*) Day-hospital and community treatment for acute psychiatric illness. A critical appraisal. *British Journal of Psychiatry*, **154**, 300–310.

——, ANTHONY, P., GODBERT, K., *et al* (1989*b*) Treatment of severe psychiatric illness in a day hospital. *British Journal of Psychiatry*, **154**, 341–437.

CREER, C., STURT, E. & WYKES, T. (1982) The role of relatives. In *Long-Term Community Care: Experience in a London Borough* (ed. J. K. Wing). Monograph suppl. *Psychological Medicine*, **2**, 29–39.

CULLBERG, J. & STEFANSSON, C. G. (1981) *An Evaluation of the Nacka Project*. Stockholm: Spri Publications.

DIBELLA, G., WEITZ, G. W., POGNTES BERGEN, D., *et al* (eds) (1982) *Handbook of Partial Hospitalisation*. New York: Brunner/Mazel.

DICKEY, B., McGUIRE, T., CANNON, N., *et al* (1986) Mental health cost models: refinements and applications. *Medical Care*, **24**, 857–866.

DORWART, R. A. (1988) A ten-year follow-up study of the effects of deinstitutionalisation. *Hospital and Community Psychiatry*, **38**, 287–291.

DOWELL, D. A. & CIARLO, J. A. (1983) Overview of the community mental health centres program from an evaluation perspective. *Community Mental Health Journal*, **19**, 95–125.

DRUMMOND, M. F., *et al* (1987) *Methods for the Economic Evaluation of Health Care Programmes*. Oxford: Oxford University Press.

EUROPEAN ECONOMIC COMMUNITY (EEC) (1981) *Evaluation and Mental Health Care: Third European Seminar on Health Policy*. Report EUR 7172. Brussels: EEC.

FENTON, R. F., TESSIER, L. & STRUENING, E. L. (1979) A comparative trial of home and hospital care. *Archives of General Psychiatry*, **36**, 1073–1079.

FORD, M., GODDARD, C. & LANSDALL-WELFARE, R. (1987) The dismantling of the mental hospital? 1960–1985 Glenside Hospital Surveys. *British Journal of Psychaitry*, **151**, 479–495.

FREEMAN, H. L., RYERS, T. & HENDERSON, J. H. (1982) *Patterns of Mental Services in Europe: 10 Years on.* Public Health in Europe no. 25. Copenhagen: WHO Regional Office for Europe.

GIEL, R. & TEN HORN, G. H. M. M. (1982) Patterns of mental health care in a Dutch register area. *Social Psychiatry*, **17**, 117–123.

GLASS, N. J. & GOLDBERG, D. (1977) Cost-benefit analysis and the evaluation of psychiatric services. *Psychological Medicine*, **7**, 701–717.

GOLDSTEIN, J. M. & HORGAN, C. M. (1988) In-patient and out-patient psychiatric services: substitutes or complements? *Hospital and Community Psychiatry*, **39**, 632–636.

GRAD, J. SAINSBURY, P. (1968) The effects that patients have on their families in a community care and a control psychiatric service. *British Journal of Psychiatry*, **114**, 265–278.

GRIFFITH, R. (1988) *Community Care: Agenda for Action.* London: HMSO.

GUDEMAN, J. E., SHORE, M. F. & DICKEY, B. (1983) Day hospitalisation and an inn instead of in-patient care for psychiatric patients. *New England Journal of Medicine*, **308**, 749–753.

GUTTENTAG, M. & STRUENING, E. L. (1975) *Handbook of Evaluation Research.* Vol. 2. Beverly Hills, California: Sage

HÄFNER, H. (1987) Do we still need beds for psychiatric patients? An analysis of changing patterns of mental health care. *Acta Psychiatrica Scandinavica*, **75**, 113–126.

—— & KLUG, J. (1982) The impact of an expanding community mental health service on patterns of bed usage: evaluation of a four-year period of implementation. *Psychological Medicine*, **12**, 177–190.

HÄFNER, H. & AN DER HEIDEN, W. (1989) The evaluation of mental health care systems. *British Journal of Psychiatry*, **155**, 12–17.

HALL, P. & BROCKINGTON, I. F. (eds) (1991) *The Closure of Mental Hospitals.* London: Gaskell.

HARE, E. H. & WING, J. K. (eds) (1970) *Psychiatric Epidemiology.* London: Oxford University Press.

HELGASON (ed.) (1983) *Methodology in Evaluation of Psychiatric Treatment.* Cambridge: Camberwell University Press.

HERZ, M. I., ENDICOTT, J., SPITZER, R. L., *et al* (1972) Day versus in-patient hospitalisation, a controlled study. *American Journal of Psychiatry*, **127**, 1371–1381.

—— (1982) Research overview in day treatment. *International Journal of Partial Hospitalisation*, **1**, 33–44.

HOLLAND, W. W. (ed.) (1983) Evaluation of Health Care. Oxford: Oxford University Press.

HOULT, J., REYNOLDS, I., CHARBONNEAU-POWIS, M., *et al* (1983) Psychiatric hospital versus community treatment: the results of a randomised trial. *Australian and New Zealand Journal of Psychiatry*, **17**, 160–267.

—— (1986) Community care of the mentally ill. *British Journal of Psychiatry*, **149**, 137–144.

HYDE, C., BRIDGES, K., GOLDBERG, D., *et al* (1987) The evaluation of a hostel ward: a controlled study using modified cost-benefit analysis. *British Journal of Psychiatry*, **151**, 805–812.

JONES, K., ROBINSON, M. & GOLIGHTLY, M. (1986) Long-term psychiatric patients in the community. *British Journal of Psychiatry*, **149**, 537–540.

KLUITER, H. (1987) *Instrument ter meting van de last op partners van psychiatrische patienten.* (ITOB: Instrument for measuring the burden of partners of psychiatric patients). Groningen: Department of Social Psychiatry, University of Groningen.

KUNZE, H. (1985) Rehabilitation and institutionalisation in community care in West Germany. *British Journal of Psychiatry*, **147**, 261–264.

LUBER, R. (ed.) (1979) *Partial Hospitalisation: A Current Perspective.* New York: Plenum.

MANGEN, S. P. (ed.) (1985) *Mental Health Care in the European Community.* London: Croom Helm.

MCCREADY, R. G., AFFLECK, J. W. & ROBINSON, A. D. (1985) The Scottish survey of psychiatric rehabilitation and support services. *British Journal of Psychiatry*, **147**, 289–294.

MCGRATH, G. & TANTAM, D. (1987) Long-stay patients in a psychiatric day hospital. *British Journal of Psychiatry*, **150**, 836–840.

MOSHER, L. R. & BURTI, L. (1989) *Community Mental Health: Principles of Practice.* New York: Norton.

MUNK-JORGENSEN, P. (1985) Cumulated need for psychiatric service as shown in a community psychiatric project. *Psychological Medicine*, **15**, 629–635.

ROSIE, J. S. (1987) Partial hospitalisation. A review of literature. *Hospital and Community Psychiatry*, **38**, 1291–1299.

SARTORIUS, N. & HARDING, T. W. (1983) Issues in the evaluation of mental health care. In *Evaluation of Health Care* (ed. W. W. Holland), pp. 243–262. Oxford: Oxford University Press.

SCHWEFEL, D., ZOLLNER, H. & POTHOFF, P. (eds) (1988) *Costs and Effects of Managing Chronic Psychotic Patients*. Berlin: Springer Verlag.

SCHENE, A. & GERSONS, B. P. R. (1986) Effectiveness and application of partial hospitalisation. *Acta Psychiatrica Scandinavica*, **74**, 335–340.

STEIN, L. I. & TEST, M. A. (1980) Alternative to mental hospital treatment. Conceptual mode, treatment program and clinical evaluation. *Archives of General Psychiatry*, **37**, 392–397.

STEINHART, I. & BOSCH, G. (1983) Development and current status of partial hospitalisation in the Federal Republic of Germany and West Berlin. *International Journal of Partial Hospitalisation*, **2**, 57–66.

STROMGREN, E., DUPONT, A. & ACHTON NIELSEN, J. (eds) (1980) *Epidemiological Research as Basis for the Organisation of Extramural Psychiatry*. Copenhagen: Munksgaard.

STRUENING, E. L. & GUTTENTAG, M. (eds) (1975) *Handbook of Evaluation Research*. Vol. 1. Beverly Hills, California: Sage

SUCHMAN, E. A. (1967) *Evaluative Research. Principles and Practice in Public Service and Social Action Programs*. New York: Russell Sage Foundation.

SYTEMA, S., GIEL, R. & TEN HORN, G. H. M. M. (1989) Patterns of care in the field of mental health. *Acta Psychiatrica Scandinavica*, **79**, 1–10.

TANSELLA, M., DE SALVIA, D. & WILLIAMS, P. (1987) The Italian psychiatric reform: some quantitative evidence. *Social Psychiatry*, **22**, 37–48.

—— & WILLIAMS, P. (1987) The Italian experience and its implications. *Psychological Medicine*, **17**, 283–289.

TANTAM, D. & MCGRATH, G. (1989) Psychiatric day hospitals – another route to institutionalisation? *Social Psychiatry and Psychiatric Epidemiology*, **24**, 96–101.

TEN HORN, G. H. M. M., GIEL, R., GULBINAT, W. H., *et al* (1986) *Psychiatric Case Registers in Public Health (1960–1985). A Worldwide Inventory*. Amsterdam: Elsevier.

THOLEN, A. J., HOEK, H. W. & GIEL, R. (1988) The classification and assessment of intellectual and other psychological impairments in the mentally disabled. *International Journal of Mental Health*, **16**, 60–77.

VAN DE POEL, J. H. R. (1986) *Judgement and Control. Individual and Organisational Aspects of Performance Evaluation*. Groningen: Wolters-Noordhoff.

VAUGHAN, P. J. (1985) Developments in psychiatric day care. *British Journal of Psychiatry*, **147**, 1–4.

WASHBRUN, S. & VANNICELLI, M. (1976) A controlled comparison of psychiatric day treatment and in-patient hospitalisation. *Journal of Consulting and Clinical Psychology*, **44**, 665–675.

WORLD HEALTH ORGANIZATION (1971) *Trends in Psychiatric Care: Day Hospitals and Units in General Hospitals*. Copenhagen: WHO Regional Office for Europe.

—— (1980) *Changing Patterns in Mental Health Care: Report on a WHO Working Group*. Copenhagen: WHO Regional Office for Europe.

—— (1986) *Mental Health Services in Southern Countries of the European Region* (EURO Reports and Studies 107). Copenhagen: WHO Regional Office for Europe.

—— (1987) *Mental Health Services in Pilot Study Areas*. Report on European Study. Copenhagen: WHO.

WIERSMA, D. (1986) Psychological impairments and social disabilities: on the applicability of the International Classification of Impairments, Disabilities and Handicaps (ICIDH) to psychiatry. *Rehabilitative Medicine*, **8**, 3–7.

——, DEJONG, A. & ORMEL, J. (1988) The Groningen Social Disabilities Schedule: development, relationship with the ICIDH, and psychometric properties. *International Journal of Rehabilitative Research*, **11**, 213–224.

—— , KLUITER, H., NIENHUIS, F. J., *et al* (1989) *Day-treatment with Community Care as an Alternative to Standard Hospitalisation: An Experiment in the Netherlands. A Preliminary Communication.* Groningen: Department of Social Psychiatry, University of Groningen.

WILLIAMS, P., WILKINSON, G. & RAWNSLEY, K. (eds) (1989) *The Scope of Epidemiological Psychiatry*. London: Routledge.

WING, J. K. (ed.) (1982) *Long-term Community Care: Experience in a London Borough.* Monograph Suppl. *Psychological Medicine*, **2**, 1–98.

—— & HAILEY, A. M. (1972) *Evaluating a Community Psychiatric Service: The Camberwell Register 1964–1971*. London: Oxford University Press.

—— , COOPER, J. E. & SARTORIUS, N. (1974) *Measurement and Classification of Psychiatric Symptoms*. London: Cambridge University Press.

WOLFF, N., HENDERSON, P. R., MACASKILL, R. L., *et al* (1989) Treatment patterns of schizophrenia in psychiatric hospitals. *Social Science and Medicine*, **28**, 323–331.

7 Do long-stay patients benefit from community placement?

JULIAN LEFF

Over the past 40 years, changes have taken place in the provision of long-term psychiatric care which have affected hundreds of thousands of patients worldwide. The decline of the mental hospital has been most dramatic in England and Wales, the USA, and Italy, although it has also occurred in other European countries. On the other hand, there are countries, for example, Japan, in which the mental hospital population still continues to expand. It is a remarkable fact that very little research has been directed at the evaluation of this revolution in the care of the chronic mentally ill. In particular, apart from a few, small-scale, follow-up studies, e.g. Jones (1985), we know of no attempt other than the Team for the Assessment of Psychiatric Services (TAPS) project to determine whether the new mode of care actually benefits the patients involved. We can speculate on the reasons for this neglect (such as reluctance to treat government policies as experiments, low scientific status of health services research), but the first priority is to remedy it. Important issues arise with respect to the design of such a study, and to the choice of research instruments.

Design issues

Ideally, one would want to set up a randomised, controlled trial in which, for a specified period of time, experimental patients were discharged to community facilities, while control patients remained in the institution. In practice, this design is most unlikely to be adopted anywhere, since research workers do not normally have sufficient control over the discharge process to insist on randomisation. This point is well illustrated by the situation that the TAPS team was faced with when setting up its central project. The North East Thames Regional Health Authority (NETRHA) decided, in July 1983, to close two of the six large mental hospitals in the region, over the course of ten years. This was seen as an opportunity to evaluate the closure policy, and after a period of negotiation, NETRHA set up TAPS to undertake this task. As the magnitude of the project became evident, TAPS grew in size, and currently comprises eight full-time research workers, with an honorary director. Funding is partly from NETRHA and partly from the Department of Health.

The two hospitals to be closed are Friern and Claybury, which between them serve nine health districts, with a total population of one million. In response to the closure decision, the health districts set up Core Teams, whose remit was to select long-term patients for discharge and to prepare them for life in the community. The Core Teams were multi-disciplinary and in almost every case led by non-psychiatrists. Thus, the discharge decisions were generally not under the control of hospital-based personnel, a fact which made it extremely unlikely that randomisation of discharges would be acceptable to the Core Teams. However, another local factor ruled out this design entirely.

In announcing the closure decision, NETRHA laid down only three guidelines for community facilities, preferring to delegate detailed planning to the district health authorities. One was that facilities should be domestic in scale, with a maximum of 24 places, but, in retrospect, this limit appears too high, as reprovision facilities for long-stay patients have so far rarely exceeded eight places. The other two stipulations have in fact had a major impact on the evaluation. One was that patients should be relocated in the community together with their friends, effectively nullifying the possibility of randomised discharges. The final policy statement was that the acute admission facilities should be the last service to be transferred from the mental hospitals. This was an enlightened decision, intended to prevent stagnation in the declining institutions; it meant that TAPS would give priority to the evaluation of long-stay, non-demented patients, since these would be discharged first.

With randomisation ruled out, the next choice is a matched case-control design. This had already been successfully employed in the evaluation by Dr Lorna Wing (Wing, 1989) of the closure of Darenth Park Hospital for the mentally handicapped. The strategy is to match each patient who is due for discharge with a patient who is likely to remain in hospital for a further year, and then to follow-up both members of the pair, a year later. However, there are a number of problems with this design. Firstly, there is the choice of variables on which to match the mover and stayer: one wants to select the factors that determine the ability to remain out of hospital, but this is a Catch 22 situation, since we shall be able to identify these only at an advanced stage of the follow-up study. At the beginning of the study, only educated guesses can be made about the factors that are likely to emerge from the data analysis as important. The variables we selected for matching on were: hospital (Friern or Claybury), age, sex, length of stay, diagnosis, and social disability. Whereas the first four variables are obtainable from hospital records, the latter two necessitate interviews with the patient, staff, or both. Thus, it was not possible to match accurately on all six factors, until we had completed a baseline assessment on all eligible patients.

Unfortunately, it took two years to complete the baseline assessments on the 770 patients in the two hospitals who met the criteria for the study. Consequently, when we began on 1 August 1985 to look for matches for patients to be discharged, we could match accurately only on the first four variables and approximately on diagnosis. We were unable to match on social disability, and much later, when the data became available, we found that the first-year cohort of discharges was significantly less disabled in social behaviour than their matches. However, by the time the second-year cohort of discharges needed matching, we not only had the data we required, but had also written a computer program that completed the matching process automatically.

Another type of problem arises from the assumptions behind the matched case-control design. These are that the courses of illness and of social disability over time, in the patients remaining in hospital, represent the 'natural history' of their conditions, albeit in an institutional setting. Any difference between the progress of discharged patients and that of their matched stayers could then be attributed to the effects of being in the community. However, as depicted in Fig. 7.1, the decision to close a mental hospital disturbs the 'natural history' of the inmates' conditions.

In situations such as this, influences of two opposing kinds operate. On the one hand, morale sinks in the declining institution. Maintenance of the fabric of the building is no longer carried out. Senior staff leave, seeing no future for themselves, while it becomes increasingly difficult to recruit junior staff. On the other hand, the staff, knowing that the remaining patients will have to be discharged if they do not die first, make increasing efforts to rehabilitate them. The net result of these two opposing trends could be either an improvement or a deterioration in a patient's condition, depending on the balance of forces. In fact, in the TAPS project, we have not recorded any significant changes in the matched patients who remained in hospital, suggesting that the opposing influences have cancelled each other out.

We have been able to find close matches for the great majority of the patients discharged in the first three years of the project. However, the pool of patients available for matching is shrinking, as more and more are discharged, and we anticipate that, by the fourth year, matching will no longer be a viable strategy. However, as we have found relative stability in the mental state and social behaviour of patients remaining in hospital, it is justifiable to use the subsequent leavers as their own controls. The assumption is that any changes detected between the baseline assessment in hospital and the follow-up in the community are attributable to life in

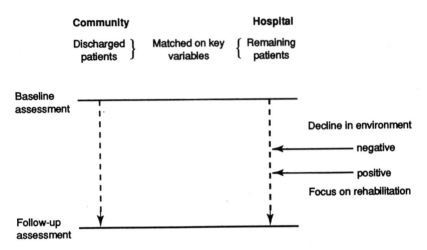

Fig. 7.1. The case-control design

the community, since, had they remained in hospital, the measures would have been unchanged.

Assessment measures

In selecting a batch of assessment instruments, we had to consider carefully the outcome criteria which were of greatest relevance to the question which initiated the research: does the policy of hospital closure benefit the patients? It was obvious that we needed to assess the mental state and social disabilities of the patients. We also felt, for the following reasons, that we should measure their physical ill-health. Firstly, we knew this to be an elderly population, with a mean age close to 60. Secondly, their physical health had been closely monitored by the nursing staff and by the junior psychiatrists who acted as their general practitioners. We were concerned that, once in the community, patients might not receive the same careful attention to their physical health. Our anxieties had been raised by several preventable deaths from physical illness of discharged long-stay patients.

In considering the issue of quality of life, we saw an imperative need to ask patients their opinion about the care they received, and to assess the degree of restrictiveness of their environment. Finally, we were concerned to chart the social networks of patients, partly to check whether they were indeed being placed in the community in company with their friends, and partly to determine whether they would develop social links with individuals in the community.

The instruments chosen for each of these areas of enquiry will next be described.

Personal Data and Psychiatric History Schedule (PDPH)

This schedule was designed to collect basic data on patients' demographic characteristics, including ethnicity, and factual information about length of stay and previous admissions. The data were collected partly from case-notes and partly from staff. Wherever possible, each patient's primary diagnosis was derived from the case-notes, but, in the course of a long admission, this had often changed several times. Where there was doubt, the patient's consultant was asked to provide a definitive diagnosis.

Present State Examination (PSE)

In view of the prominent negative symptoms to be expected in this population, we first used the Krawiecka scale (Krawiecka *et al*, 1977) in a pilot study. However, in our hands, this did not yield satisfactory levels of inter-rater reliability. We therefore chose to use the PSE, particularly as it has been employed in so many studies, both national and international. We were conscious of the problem posed by patients who deny psychotic symptoms in response to the PSE, but who are well known by nursing staff to harbour florid delusions or to regularly converse with auditory hallucinations. To accommodate this, we added two items which record information from the nursing staff about active psychotic symptoms when the patient denies them.

Physical Health Index (PHI)

We did not have enough medically qualified research staff to examine each patient physically. Instead, we derived information from case-notes and from the ward staff. The information was collected with respect to seven bodily systems, for each of which two ratings were made: the level of disability and the level of medical or nursing care received. In addition, problems with incontinence, immobility, and dyskinesia were noted, as these are likely to hinder community placement.

Social Behaviour Schedule (SBS)

We used this schedule, developed in the unit by Wykes & Sturt (1986), which is of established reliability. However, when we began interviewing discharged patients with it, we became aware of some gaps in the schedule. These were mostly to do with areas of self-care which patients were allowed little or no opportunity to exercise in hospital. We needed to develop a supplementary

D

schedule to cover these areas, but this could not be given to all patients in the hospital cohort, because of the stage at which the deficiency in the SBS was noticed. The additional schedule is known as Basic Everyday Living Skills (BELS) and is now in a final form, after piloting, but is currently undergoing reliability tests. Both schedules rely on information given by staff.

Environmental Index (EI)

This schedule was developed from instruments existing in the unit, and measures the degree of restrictiveness of the patient's environment. In that respect, it reflects institutional practices. We added some questions on the accessibility of a variety of amenities which would be important for patients in the community. These include shops, launderettes, pubs, parks, and day centres or day hospitals.

Patient Attitude Questionnaire (PAQ)

Patients are asked what they like or dislike about their current caring environment. There are also questions about their desire to leave hospital or to stay, and about where they would prefer to live.

Social Network Schedule (SNS)

We constructed this questionnaire *ab initio*, as nothing suitable existed. The inquiry begins with the completion of a time budget, providing the context of activity within which social contacts are made. All the people named by the patient constitute his or her social universe. Within this, he is asked to identify which individuals he talks to regularly, who would be missed if not seen, whom he would visit if they were separated, who is considered to be a friend, and whom he would confide in.

Initially, we employed two versions of this schedule – one for patients and one for staff to give information about patients. It soon became evident, however, that staff overestimated the number of friends that patients had on the ward and knew little or nothing about their social contacts off the ward. Consequently, we stopped collecting these data from staff, even though it meant having no SNS information for patients who refused or were unable to complete the interview.

Use of community facilities

For discharged patients, information was collected on the use of community facilities, such as day centres, CPNs, and GPs, to enable the economists to calculate the cost of all the services which were provided to replace the psychiatric hospital.

Collection of the full batch of information occupied about half a day per patient. We began by drawing up a list of patients in the two hospitals who met the criteria for inclusion in the cohort, viz. a continuous stay in hospital of more than one year, and no evidence of dementia if aged over 65. We included all patients under 65, even if they had dementia, since they would be considered for reprovision alongside the non-demented. At the start of assessments, in August 1985, the cohort comprised about 900 patients, but more than 100 of the older patients died before they could be interviewed. Assessments were in fact carried out on a total of 770 patients, of whom 373 were in Friern and 397 in Claybury, and took two years to complete.

Data management and analysis

It has to be appreciated that a sample of 1000 patients, interviewed on at least two occasions, with a batch of instruments including 500 items, generates one million bits of information. There are huge problems involved in managing such a massive data set, and in organising and conducting its analysis. A project of this magnitude needs advice on data handling from the beginning, as well as the services of an expert in computing and statistics.

Early in the TAPS project, considerable pressure was exerted on us by planning teams to provide them with our baseline assessment data, which were seen to be of great value in assisting the planning process. We felt it was important for us to respond to the requests for data, as this would probably reinforce the cooperation of clinical staff, on whom we relied to complete our interviews. Therefore, we prepared clinical feedback forms on each patient we interviewed, and made these available to the responsible clinical team, but excluded data that were collected from the patient under conditions of confidentiality, i.e. data from the Patient Attitude Questionnaire and the Social Network Schedule.

Sociological study

In addition to the central project, which is essentially clinical in nature, a sociological study is being conducted of the processes of decision-making which lead to implementation of new services and facilities (Tomlinson, 1988). The sociologists involved in this research attend planning meetings as observers, but make no contribution to the meetings themselves. However, they do interview key participants before or afterwards, to clarify issues about decision-making. They cover the whole hierarchy of meetings, from the regional management down to case conferences about individual patients.

The value of this work lies in its comparative nature. It is possible to compare health districts with different political leadership, with differing styles of management, and with varying success rates in achieving the goals of implementation. This is likely to identify those management structures and policies which lead to success in providing facilities alternative to the mental hospital.

Economic study

In these times of particular financial stringency, it is clearly of great importance to calculate the cost of the community services that are designed to replace the mental hospitals. This is no easy matter, since patients are being discharged to a wide variety of facilities – statutory, voluntary, and private. Furthermore, many different sources of funding are used to support patients discharged into the community. One crucial innovation in the Friern–Claybury reprovision is to attach to each discharged patient the annual revenue that it costs to maintain the patient in hospital: this currently amounts to about £14 000 per annum. This revenue goes to the district health authority which accepts responsibility for the discharged patients, and remains in their budget even after the patient has died. Since many of the Friern and Claybury long-stay patients are elderly, this represents a strong incentive for health authorities to make provisions for them and to ensure that they remain in the district's care.

What has become the commonest form of community provision for these patients also represents an innovation. It consists of an ordinary house, bought either by the health authority or a voluntary organisation, and converted for the use of from 3 to 12 patients. Nursing staff and other professionals may be present in the house for up to 24 hours a day, depending on the level of disability of the patients. The most intensive staffing levels used to date represent a staff–patient ratio of 1 : 1, which is comparable with that of an acute admission ward. The costs of staffing such homes are, of course, included in the overall economic calculations, and, as a result, accommodation and living expenses occupy over 75% of the cost of community care for these patients.

The cost of hospital care is also not simple to estimate, since an average that is derived by dividing the total annual budget by the number of patients fails to take into account the great variation in costs incurred by different groups of patients. For example, the cost of an acute admission ward with a high staffing level is much greater than that of a long-stay ward, which has small numbers of staff, as well as patients who may be contributing to the income of the hospital by their work in industrial therapy. In order to take due account of this variation, it is necessary to disaggregate hospital costs, at least down to a ward level, and in some instances to an individual patient level.

In the TAPS project, the team of economists has worked very closely with the clinical research workers, in order that the characteristics of individual patients in each cohort can be related to their service usage. It then becomes possible to make predictions about the cost of community care for patients who are still in hospital but will eventually be discharged. This kind of calculation showed that one can account for 36% of the variance in the cost of community care for discharged patients by using their characteristics at baseline assessment, while they were still in-patients. This is a surprisingly high proportion, and lends some confidence to the notion of prediction of future costs for patients not yet discharged (Knapp *et al*, 1990).

Specific problems in the Friern–Claybury reprovision

Accumulation of new long-stay patients

Our census of the long-stay non-demented patients in the two hospitals began on 31 August 1985: any patient whose stay in hospital exceeded one year after that date and who qualified in other ways for our study, joined the study population. However, a distinction was made between patients qualifying on the census date – the base population – and those entering the study thereafter – accumulation patients. The accumulation rates are monitored on a monthly basis, since they have a vital bearing on the run-down of the hospitals. It soon became evident that the two hospitals, although containing very similar populations of patients in many respects, had quite different accumulation rates. Although Claybury serves a larger catchment population than does Friern (550 000, as opposed to 450 000), its accumulation rate is much lower. Over the three years between August 1985 and August 1988, the total number of accumulation patients at Friern was 164 (Margolius, 1988), compared with 69 at Claybury.

This was a puzzling difference, which initially was thought to be possibly attributable to the higher number of homeless patients and patients from outside the catchment area who are admitted to Friern. However, very few such individuals were actually found among either the Claybury or Friern accumulation. Another line of inquiry was pursued by comparing the accumulation rate for each health district with its Jarman Index – the relative ranking of an area in terms of a composite of measures of social deprivation (Jarman, 1984). A working party of the Royal College of Psychiatrists (1988) had already established that there was a close relationship between the use of psychiatric beds as a whole and the Jarman Index. Table 7.1 displays the rates of accumulation and Jarman Index ranking for the health districts served by Friern and Claybury.

It can be seen that the accumulation rate for each of the Friern districts is higher than that for any of the Claybury districts. There is a strikingly high association between the accumulation rates and the Jarman Index

TABLE 7.1
Accumulation rates and Jarman Index ranking for nine health districts

Health district	Accumulation rate per 100 000	Jarman Index
Friern Hospital		
Hampstead	2.5	18
Bloomsbury	3.8	9
Islington	4.3	8
West Haringey	3.4	55
Claybury Hospital		
Waltham Forest	1.5	40
Redbridge	0.7	161
East Haringey	1.9	15
Enfield/Edmonton	0.5	104
West Essex	0.8	178

Spearman's rank order correlation between accumulation rate and Jarman Index = 0.82.

rankings (R = 0.82). This suggests that social deprivation in the catchment population is a major determinant of the accumulation rate.

This has obvious importance for reprovision, since the higher the rate of accumulation of new long-stay patients, the slower the run-down of long-stay beds in the hospital. Furthermore, we have found that the accumulation patients make up a disproportionate amount of the discharges from long-stay beds at Friern. Thus, in the first three years of discharges from Friern, accumulation patients occupied 22%, 46%, and 49%, respectively, of the cohorts, while the corresponding proportions for Claybury were 0%, 6%, and 14%. As a result, there has been a smaller reduction in the number of the base population at Friern than at Claybury – 20% compared with 31%. Furthermore, different types of community provision are required by the accumulation patients, since they are significantly younger than baseline patients, have a much shorter cumulative length of hospital stay, and are significantly less likely to carry a diagnosis of schizophrenia.

Although this may be a local peculiarity, the link between long-stay accumulation and social deprivation suggests that the latter is likely to be an important factor in any attempt to close psychiatric hospitals serving inner-city areas, and in the evaluation of such a process.

Creaming-off

It is understandable that the teams selecting patients for discharge should choose the least disabled first. However, this practice has profound consequences both for the process of reprovision and for its evaluation. The way in which creaming-off has affected the discharges from Friern and Claybury differentially is shown in Table 7.2.

For the first three years of discharges from Claybury, there is a progressive increase in the mean age, duration of stay, and number of problems in social behaviour from year to year. This progression is not evident for Friern

TABLE 7.2

Characteristics of three consecutive cohorts of leavers from Friern and Claybury hospitals and the remaining patients

Year	No. (accumulation)		Mean age: years	Mean years in hospital	Median SBS score
Claybury Hospital					
1	12	(0)	54.2	17.3	0
2	48	(3)	55.5	20.1	2.5
3	58	(8)	56.6	23.2	4.5
Remaining 305			61.0	27.4	6
Friern Hospital					
1	32	(7)	54.3	7.8	2
2	72	(33)	49.7	12.4	4
3	63	(31)	54.8	11.8	3
Remaining 324			58.3	22.2	6

discharges, however, because it has been masked by the high proportion of accumulation patients in the second- and third-year cohorts. Of course, this in itself represents a differential selection of the least disabled since, as reported above, accumulation patients are younger, have been in hospital a shorter time, and have a lower proportion of schizophrenics than does the base population.

The consequences for reprovision include escalating difficulties for hospital staff as they try to rehabilitate an increasingly disabled group of remaining patients, and the need for community planners to develop new types of facilities for these residual patients. Facilities that work reasonably well for the first few cohorts of discharges may be inappropriate for the most disabled patients still in hospital. Many of the remainder appear from our SNS data to be completely asocial, and we have grave doubts as to their ability to form cohesive social groups, when placed in homes in the community.

The effects of creaming-off on evaluative research are equally momentous. It can be seen from Table 7.2 that even by the third year of discharges, the patients in the cohort are less disadvantaged on each measure than those remaining in hospital. As a result, neither the results of the clinical follow-up of this cohort, nor of the economic analysis, can be extrapolated to the patients still to be discharged. Although a high accumulation rate may not be found in other hospitals undergoing closure, it is inevitable that creaming-off will occur unless there is an explicit policy contravening it. Therefore, our warning against drawing premature conclusions from the study of the first few years of discharges will apply.

Preliminary findings of the TAPS project

The baseline assessments were completed after two years, and comprised 397 patients at Claybury and 373 at Friern. A comparison of the samples from the two hospitals revealed very few significant differences on any of the schedules, suggesting that patients with similar characteristics have been left behind in psychiatric hospitals after four decades of an active discharge policy (NETRHA, 1988). The one-year and two-year follow-ups have been completed and a preliminary analysis of the data carried out. In the first year from August 1985, 44 patients were discharged from the two hospitals, mostly to private care homes. In the second year, the majority of the 117 patients discharged went to purpose-planned group homes. Only three patients were lost to follow-up and probably drifted into vagrancy, which had been their previous lifestyle; no patient went to prison or committed suicide. There were four deaths in the second-year cohort of discharges and the same number in the matched group. A handful of patients were charged with minor criminal offences. In all, 29 patients were readmitted to hospital during the follow-up period, most of whom were discharged back to the community.

Analysis of the data derived from the follow-up interviews revealed that very few significant changes over time had affected discharged patients differentially from their matches. The three main effects over time were that the leavers were living in a much less restrictive environment than previously, that they were much more content with their living situation than they had been in hospital, and that they viewed their medication as much less helpful than previously. The latter change is hard to interpret, but the first two are a tribute to deinstitutionalisation. However, there were no significant changes in the patients' mental states, social disabilities, or social networks. A two-year follow-up, which is being conducted on discharged patients, may detect further beneficial changes over time. The surprising finding from the economic analysis was that community care for the first two cohorts of discharges was less costly than care in hospital. We have already cautioned against extrapolating these findings to the more disabled patients remaining in hospital.

Conclusions

An enormous expenditure of time and effort has been invested in the TAPS project. This is appropriate, because no previous study has attempted a comprehensive evaluation of the policy of closing psychiatric hospitals. It would certainly be desirable for projects on a similar scale to be mounted in other countries in which this policy is being pursued, but it is probably unrealistic to expect this. A reasonable compromise would be to dispense with the matched control group of patients remaining in hospital. This can be supported on two grounds: firstly, that this design is viable only for the first few years of discharges, and secondly, that we found no significant changes over time which affected the matched patients.

Concentrating solely on discharged patients saves a great deal of effort, since it is then unnecessary to assess the whole baseline population. Instead, patients selected for discharge are assessed while in hospital, and again at follow-up; they thus act as their own controls. An economic analysis can also be applied to these patients, by calculating the cost of their hospital care before discharge and comparing it with their cost in the community. A study with this design should be feasible in any European country.

References

JARMAN, B. (1984) Underprivileged areas: validation and distribution of scores. *British Medical Journal*, **289**, 1587–1592.
JONES, K. (1985) *After Hospital: A Study of Long-term Psychiatric Patients in York.* York: University of York/York Health Authority.
KNAPP, M., BEECHAM, S., ANDERSON, J., *et al* (1990) The TAPS project 3: Predicting the costs of closing psychiatric hospitals. *British Journal of Psychiatry*, **157**, 661–670.
KRAWIECKA, M., GOLDBERG, D. & VAUGHAN, M. (1977) A standardised psychiatric assessment schedule for rating psychiatric patients. *Acta Psychiatrica Scandinavica*, **55**, 299–308.
NORTH EAST THAMES REGIONAL HEALTH AUTHORITY (1988) *Team for the Assessment of Psychiatric Services: Preliminary Report on Baseline Data from Friern and Claybury Hospitals.* London: NETRHA.
MARGOLIUS, O. (1988) *Friern Hospital 1985–1988: Movement and Accumulation of the Long-stay Population.* London: NETRHA.
ROYAL COLLEGE OF PSYCHIATRISTS (1988) *Psychiatric Beds and Resources: Factors Influencing Bed Use and Service Planning.* Report of a Working Party. London: Gaskell.
TOMLINSON, D. (1988) *The Administrative Process of Claybury and Friern Reprovision.* London: NETRHA.
WING, L. (1989) *Hospital Closure and the Resettlement of Residents.* Aldershot: Avebury (Gower Publishing Group).
WYKES, T. & STURT, E. (1986) The measurement of social behaviour in psychiatric patients: an assessment of the reliability and validity of the SBS schedule. *British Journal of Psychiatry*, **148**, 1–11.

Discussion (some comments on the study population, design, and methods): RAIMO K. R. SALOKANGAS

The discharge of psychiatric patients from hospital to the community can have either positive or negative consequences – for the patients themselves, for their relatives, and for society at large. The outcome of the process depends on a wide range of both individual and community factors.

The key factor in the decision to discharge mentally ill patients is their social capacity or any shortcomings in that capacity (social disablement; Wing & Morris, 1981). If community placement is to benefit patients, they must possess a minimum level of social skills, as well as be able to tolerate pressure and meet reasonable demands imposed by the environment. These essential skills, which may either never have developed in the patient or which may have been lost in the course of the illness, can be acquired or recovered through rehabilitation. However, good social capacity is not enough in itself; discharged long-stay patients also need a comprehensive support system which can provide them with social support (housing, social interaction, and activity), keep up the rehabilitation process, alleviate related stress factors, and generally help patients cope with the pressures and difficulties which are bound to develop.

Some criteria of successful community placement

Discharge from hospital can be described as a positive change and as beneficial for patients when this gives them increased freedom of action, in comparison with life n hospital, means an improvement in their overall quality of life; and reduces the problems typically related to hospital life, such as lack of stimulation and social interaction. However, successful discharge requires that the demands imposed on patients by life in the community do not exceed their tolerance and do not cause their clinical state to deteriorate. It is also essential that discharge from hospital does not cause unreasonable inconvenience and stress to those in patients' immediate environment – above all to their relatives – or a financial or other burden to society exceeding that caused by their treatment in hospital.

All of these criteria should be taken into consideration in evaluating the success and usefulness of placing a long-stay psychiatric patient in the community. However, this may prove to be an extremely difficult task: in the first place, it is not at all easy to measure all the above-mentioned criteria, and, secondly, these criteria are not directly comparable with each other. In the case of an individual patient, certain changes may be positive and others negative, making it quite difficult to form a clear opinion on the utility of community placement, in comparison with continued stay in hospital.

Planning a study for long-stay patients

Any study concerned with investigating psychiatric long-stay patients has to pay special attention to the definition of the basic population and to the sampling procedure, as well as the research design and methods.

Study population

In sampling long-stay patients, we can start either from the patient population of certain hospitals or from a certain catchment area and all hospitalised patients who come from that area. Since the hospitals and health care systems of the areas (or countries) involved in the study may differ considerably, the latter may be a better starting-point. This would mean including in the study not only long-stay patients, but also those cared for by the entire health care system used by the area's population.

Study design

As far as the design is concerned, perhaps the most feasible strategy is to follow the patients' movement within the care system, as well as changes in their status which occur without any (or at least only minimum) intervention in the activities of the system itself. Another possible approach is to do an intervention study which aims to influence the kind of treatment received by the patients, although, in many respects, this latter alternative is more demanding and also apparently more expensive. It might come into question after the less demanding first alternative has been tested – which is not to say that it does not involve theoretical and practical problems of its own.

As Professor Leff has pointed out, a randomised, controlled trial is very unlikely to be carried out, because of the many practical difficulties involved. The same applies to the matched case-control design, where the strategy is to match each patient who is likely to be discharged against one who is likely to remain in hospital. Such problems were obvious in a project carried out in the hospital of which I was in charge, when we looked at the effects of the ward environment on the clinical state and social capacity of long-stay patients. Thirty long-stay patients were admitted to a newly renovated ward, and matched with patients from other long-stay wards on the variables of age, sex, length of treatment, and diagnosis. The intention was to follow up the patients for a period of six months, during which they were examined three times. However, turnover and discharge rates were so high that only six couples could be successfully followed up for the whole six-month period.

In other words, the investigators are not generally in a position to control changes of wards or the discharge of patients: at least some of the control patients may be discharged during follow-up, and the probability of this happening increases if social capacity is used as a criterion in matching. In ethical terms, too, it is a dubious practice to keep control patients in hospital, if their functional status is good enough to warrant discharge. Therefore, the research project now under discussion should probably adopt a policy of minimal interference in the activities of the care systems investigated, with attention directed primarily at following their 'natural' flow of work.

Nevertheless, it might still be useful to have control cases, because every research project always has some effect on the activity of the care system. In the project in which we examined the experience of a renovated ward, although we had no intention of influencing the ward's activities, it was obvious that the nursing staff had started to pay much more attention than usual to the patients' social skills. This was one of the side-effects of our project: the nursing staff learned to analyse their patients' behaviour and actions, and found shortcomings in them that they had not noticed before. As a result of this, the patients' social capacity seemed to decline on average between the two first interviews (which were conducted by outside researchers), but then returned to its baseline level or even improved, by the time of the third measurement.

Another reason the use of control groups might be useful is that there are broad differences among the countries taking part in this project, in terms of how far they have reduced the number of their psychiatric hospital beds. This may cause considerable differences in the results, even if the length of the patients' hospital stay is controlled. There are also major differences between countries in practices of care, as well as in the availability of alternative services. Since it is clearly impossible to control all the factors that have a bearing on a patient's successful discharge, it seems that to achieve better comparability, we should include in the samples from each research area a control group of in-patients with relatively severe handicaps, who would be followed up in the same way as the cohorts of discharged patients.

Rather than matching the patients in the control groups with those who are discharged in the same area, the former would consist of the comparable groups of seriously ill, long-stay patients in all study areas. By following their movement within the care system, it should be possible, at least in principle, to examine the differences in the care practices of different areas; in turn, this would give valuable information for the explanation of possible areal differences between discharged cohorts.

Thus, it would seem useful to look into the possibilities of a study design where each research area is represented by two cohorts of patients. The first would consist of successive long-stay patients who are discharged from hospital, using relatively loose criteria for inclusion in the sample (e.g. age, length of hospital stay, and diagnosis). The second cohort would consist of long-stay in-patients who meet a stricter set of criteria (e.g. age, length of hospital stay, diagnosis, clinical state, social capacity).

Both cohorts would receive an extensive medical examination and standardised psychiatric interview in hospital; in the case of the first cohort, these would take place before discharge. This baseline investigation would also include interviews with the nursing staff and possibly with the relatives of those patients who are discharged.

Additionally, data would be collected from case records on the patients' histories of treatment and illness.

The baseline investigation would determine each patient's earlier psychiatric treatment; behaviour in treatment; attitudes towards treatment and discharge; clinical, physical, and psychiatric state; social skills; and network of human relations. It would also be necessary to look into the environment to which the patients are moving, as well as the attitudes of their relatives towards their being discharged. The investigation of the second cohort would not need to be quite as detailed.

Both cohorts would be followed up for at least one year and preferably two, with the collection of detailed information on each patient's use of health care and other services (primary health care, psychiatric care, and social services, both public and private) throughout the follow-up period. After this period (i.e. 12 or 24 months) all patients would be interviewed again. In addition, the persons responsible for their care and possibly the patients' relatives would also be interviewed. All interviews would use essentially the same scheme as at baseline.

Outside the study design, a separate investigation could be carried out of those patients who return to hospital during the follow-up period. Here, the aim would be to identify the reasons for the relapse and the factors on which services should concentrate, in trying to prevent this from happening. For the purpose of comparative analysis, data should also be collected on the availability of both social and health care services in each study area, as well as on various socio-economic factors (e.g. housing situation and level of unemployment).

Methods and study instruments

The evaluation methods used in the TAPS project could provide a useful starting-point, although there are a few problems that must first be resolved. Firstly, different countries have different diagnostic practices and even different diagnostic systems. As from the beginning of 1987, Finland adopted a new disease classification which is based on DSM–III–R, whereas other European countries still use the ICD system. However, it should not be too difficult to agree on a common diagnostic practice.

There are various methods available for the evaluation of patients' clinical state; these include the BPRS, the CPRS, the PSE, etc. In a national schizophrenia project in Finland, we followed up 227 new schizophrenic patients for a period of five years (National Board of Health, 1988). The doctors who were responsible for the treatment of these patients performed a clinical examination, and on that basis, completed the CPRS, which proved to be a reliable and useful instrument. This method has been quite popular, especially in the Scandinavian countries. The PSE is perhaps the most widely used standardised instrument for the evaluation of clinical state, and has also been used successfully in international research projects (e.g. the WHO Schizophrenia Pilot Study). This instrument requires of its user a special training, which should not be too difficult (or very expensive) to arrange from outside, in areas where there are not enough researchers who are familiar with the method. In Finland, there are researchers who have a training in this method as well as the resources to provide training for newcomers; access to the CATEGO program is also available at the National Pensions Institute.

The study should pay special attention to the physical health and health behaviour of long-stay patients. If possible, a trained doctor should evaluate the physical health of every subject at baseline, on the basis of full medical and laboratory examinations, while changes in physical condition should also be monitored during the follow-up. The follow-up of side-effects caused by neuroleptic drugs would appear to be particularly important, because there might be unexpectedly high numbers of sudden deaths among users of certain neuroleptic drugs. It is possible that, in some cases, discharge from hospital will mean lowered standards in the medical treatment and monitoring of long-stay psychiatric patients.

The evaluation of social skills and behaviour is usually based on reports by the nursing staff. However, as some of the patients are transferred to their own homes or to other forms of accommodation where there are no trained personnel, the evaluation of social skills may become quite unreliable or be altogether absent.

In our own study of out-patients with functional psychosis (Salokangas *et al*, 1991*a*,*b*), in which we used the support schedule described by Creer *et al* (1982), considerable discrepancies were found between the patients' and relatives' assessments of the degree of disturbance in the patients' social behaviour; also, the patients gave consistently higher ratings of their function in the self-care area than did their relatives. We are currently looking into this problem in the case of discharged schizophrenic patients, using the same method. As well as the patients themselves, we are also interviewing their nearest relatives and their therapists, who in most cases are staff at the community mental health centre, whom the patient visits once every four to eight weeks. Our preliminary observations indicate that the therapists do not always have a very clear picture of their patients' social skills or of their shortcomings in that area. Therefore, we need an instrument that can give reliable measurements of patients' social behaviour, both in the hospital environment and in the community.

Although Europe forms a fairly homogeneous area in cultural terms, there may still be certain differences between the study areas that will cause difficulty in making standardised assessments of the patients' quality of life and living environment. The patients' attitude to the treatment they receive and to their living environment represent important criteria of the quality of life. In addition to these, however, it might be useful to have other indicators, particularly to assess restrictive factors in the environment. A patient's social network can be evaluated in many different ways. In our national schizophrenia project, the interviewer asked patients how often during the past month they had met various people: spouses, children, parents, brothers and sisters, colleagues, neighbours, friends, other patients, nursing staff, etc. In the study of patients with functional psychosis (Salokangas *et al*, 1991*a*,*b*), we used the same method and discovered that, here, the patients themselves and their relatives gave fairly consistent assessments of the frequency of social contacts.

In our ongoing study of discharged schizophrenic patients, the same battery of questions concerning human contacts is presented to patients, to their relatives, and to therapists. At the same time, our aim is to establish the quality of those contacts by asking whether the subjects have close friends or other persons whom they can trust and turn to in their moments of despair, and what is their membership of various social communities. On this basis, the ultimate aim is to find out how the quantity and quality of human contacts between patients and near relatives differs from the social network of the therapists, with whom we are comparing our subjects. In the light of our experiences so far, there is no difficulty in establishing the number of social contacts between patients and their relatives by interview; the assessment of the quality of those contacts, however, may be far more problematic.

Special attention should be given to the careful evaluation of treatment after discharge. The problem here is that care practices and systems tend to vary across different countries. However, during follow-up, the following, at least, should be evaluated: use of neuroleptic drugs (doses and regular administration), the continuity of care and changes in the care relationship, the treatment of crisis situations, and patients' own experiences of treatment received.

The 'failures' who have had to return to hospital could be examined separately by interviewing not only the patient, but also the staff involved in treatment, and possibly the relatives. This might help to point to the factors which lie behind the unfortunate relapse and failure of community placement. At least in the initial stages, if no standardised methods are available, this investigation could form an independent sub-study of its own, using non-standardised data collection.

Any assessment of the success and usefulness of community placement of psychiatric patients must take into consideration the related financial issues. In particular, attention has to be given to the costs caused to society at large, as well as to patients and possibly their relatives. As far as the costs of hospital treatment and of other institutional care are concerned, it should be relatively easy to produce reasonably accurate estimates; the same applies to other benefits coming from the state budget, such as pensions, housing allowances, etc. On the other hand, it will be far more difficult to produce accurate calculations of the changes caused in the patient's personal budget by discharge. Given the major differences in the social security systems of different countries, it might prove necessary to have an economist on each research team.

Conclusion

The starting-points for the analysis of successful community placement of long-stay psychiatric patients have been discussed here, and a research design which may be suitable for a comparative European project described. In the proposed design, each area samples two patient cohorts, one of which consists of patients discharged from hospital and the other of hospital in-patients with severe social disabilities. Both cohorts are followed up for 1–2 years. In hospital, the investigation includes the collection of data from medical records, examination of the patient's physical and mental state, and evaluation of social capacity, social network, living environment, and quality of life. Follow-up studies are carried out 12 and 24 months after the baseline investigation: detailed data are collected on the use of social and health care services, as well as on changes in the patient's personal budget. A separate analysis should be done to determine the causes of return to hospital.

References

CREER, C., STURT, E. & WYKES, T. (1982) The role of relatives. In Long-term community care: experience in a London borough. *Psychological Medicine*, Monograph supplement, **2**, 29–39.

NATIONAL BOARD OF HEALTH (1988) *The Schizophrenia Project 1981–1987. Final Report of the National Programme for the Study, Treatment and Rehabilitation of Schizophrenic Patients in Finland.* English summary. Series Handbooks no. 4. Helsinki: National Board of Health in Finland.

SALOKANGAS, R. K. R., PALO-OJA, T. & OJANEN, M. (1991a) The need for social support among out-patients suffering from functional psychosis. *Psychological Medicine*, **27**, 209–217.

———, ———, ———, *et al* (1991b) Need for community care among psychiatric out-patients suffering from functional psychosis. *Acta Psychiatrica Scandinavica* (in press).

WING, J. K. & MORRIS, B. (1981) Clinical basis of rehabilitation. In *Handbook of Psychiatric Rehabilitation Practice*, (eds J. K. Wing & B. Morris), pp. 3–16. Oxford: Oxford University Press.

8 Improving the social competence of the chronic mentally ill

HANS D. BRENNER, MILKA MAURER and MARCO C. G. MERLO

Mental disability can be understood only if it is considered as part of the broader problem of disability *per se*. While specific areas of functioning are impaired, the entire human being is also affected. In addition, no one biological, cognitive, psychological, or emotional factor is ever the sole cause of any psychological dysfunction. Nor does any particular psychiatric illness *per se* determine the way disability is manifested. Mental disability is just as much the result of people's way of life, their social behaviour, and the society they are part of. It must, therefore, be treated both pragmatically and comprehensively.

However, the detection and identification of mental disability is not easy for lay persons, or even for the staff of mental health services. The anti-psychiatry movement succeeded in making the problem seem harmless and trivial ("from bad care to good cure"), but this movement is not alone to blame for this. Patients' organisations which claim that there are no chronic psychiatric patients, but only psychiatric 'clients' who could easily participate in normal community living, have also had a counter-productive effect on the quality of care of the mentally disabled. Finally, chronic mentally ill patients in nursing homes are overlooked even more frequently, because they do not figure in statistics of the mentally ill.

Although schizophrenic patients tend to be more seriously disabled than those with affective disorders or severe anxiety states (Harrow *et al*, 1978), almost half have to be readmitted within one year of release (Bellack *et al*, 1984), and more than 75% of chronic patients do not manage to stay out of hospital for more than three years (Falloon *et al*, 1981). Most chronically ill patients function inadequately or inappropriately in their personal and social lives (Sylph *et al*, 1978), and those who had poor social skills before discharge from hospital have significantly more relapses (Linn *et al*, 1980). The unemployment rate of the chronically mentally ill is 70% or more (Goldstrom & Manderscheid, 1982): fewer than 30% of patients have a job after leaving psychiatric hospitals, and only 10–15% manage to hold steady employment for a period of one to five years (Anthony *et al*, 1984). A majority of patients in 'nursing home' accommodation are unemployed and unmarried, and are members of the lower social classes (Shadish & Bootzin, 1984).

However, the mentally ill do not just manifest behavioural traits that are characteristic of their disorders. Frey (1984) defined mental disability from a disabled person's point of view as a "limitation to perform tasks expected of an individual within a social environment". Anthony & Liberman (1986), following WHO criteria, divided the relevant dysfunctions into three subcategories: impairment, disability, and handicap. These authors agree that, basically, the mentally ill demonstrate deficient and inappropriate behaviour that might just as well be manifested by well adjusted individuals. There is, however, a key difference: even if healthy persons do show certain behavioural disturbances or deficiencies, they are still able to lead a fulfilling and independent life in the community. Mentally ill people, on the other hand, are overwhelmed by personal problems, and are unable to deal with them; the problems are out of control. In addition to clinical symptoms, attentional/perceptual, cognitive, and emotional disorders are more severe than in other people, occur more frequently, and are interrelated. They can result in conflict situations which make successful interactions difficult. "Work tolerance, endurance, following instructions, cooperating with coworkers and supervisors, problem solving, task orientation and ability to accept criticism and ask for assistance are all examples of disabilities that are caused by symptomatic and cognitive impairments and that lead to significant handicap" (Anthony & Liberman, 1986).

On the other hand, such conflict situations are not only caused by patients' inappropriate and inadequate behaviour, but are also the result of behaviour directed towards patients in the social environment (e.g. family, job, recreational groups). The people a patient relates to may be incapable of coping with either the patient's or their own maladjusted behaviour. They suffer under the patient's or their own impairments and deficiencies and the consequences of these. Gruenberg (1969) described this phenomenon as the "social breakdown syndrome", consisting of suicidal and aggressive behaviour, poor personal hygiene, neglected family responsibilities, unemployment, etc.

From the individual point of view, 'mental disability' means difficulty in leading an independent life – one that brings reasonable subjective and objective satisfaction – within the confines of society. The concept, therefore, is directly related to individuals' social competence and to the society they belong to. In contrast to the concept of physical disability, 'mental disability' refers not only to the way individuals function, but also to the demands that certain situations make on them and to the problem situations that have to be coped with. It is revealed by patients' inability to fulfil role-demands and social expectations, representing the social aspect of mental disability.

Social competence

Research on social skills has been conducted by both social and natural scientists. According to O'Malley (1977),

> "at least three research perspectives on social competence can be identified. First is the ethological view that social competence consists of adaptive interactions in the natural environment. . . . A second view constitutes competence in the framework of structural theory of personality that attempts to integrate descriptive features of behaviours underlying purposive interactions. The final view analyzes competence in terms of social theories of behaviours underlying purposive interactions".

Thus, the concept of social competence should define to what extent certain behaviour is acceptable in a particular environment.

The numerous factors which comprise social competence can be evaluated and described at the various levels of individual and social organisation. They include both micro- and macromolecular processes in the metabolism of the neural system, neurophysiological processes, psychological processes, human relationships, and the macrosocial structure. However, what is meant, above all, by social competence, depends on the psychological and social organisational level of every social group and culture. Each one of these requires a certain number of respective behavioural patterns – 'social skills' – to be manifested. But these social skills are only some of the components of whatever forms of social competence an individual might be able to acquire. Lévi-Strauss' (1945) analysis of the acquisition of language is an analogous example. Therefore, the individual's realistic chances of acquiring social skills and of implementing them in a particular situation need to be considered with regard to the presence of any mental disability.

In terms of components of behaviour, social competence is made up of those social skills which an individual utilises to fulfil role-expectations and to perform adequately in everyday life. Those same skills also help both individuals and the groups to which they belong to survive in a constantly changing environment. On the whole, researchers agree that both the desirable and the undesirable behavioural components of social competence have been acquired through learning processes.

Social skills

Although there is no generally accepted interdisciplinary definition of 'social skills', it would be a boon for research as well as for therapeutic practice if we had one because, as Wallace *et al* (1980) have pointed out, "different conceptual definitions result in different methods of training and evaluation". Both exchange of information and evaluation of research results are made even more difficult by the fact that only a handful of authors have clearly explained what they actually mean by the term. Although systematic assessments have been made of various definitions, none have been given worldwide recognition. However, the respective definitions by Wallace *et al* (1980) and by Liberman (1982) of social competence have been very useful in our own work.

> "Social skills include affective, cognitive and motoric domains of functioning. They comprise the transactions between people that result in attainment of tangible and social-emotional goals. Skills must be demonstrated in a large variety of interpersonal contexts and require the coordinated delivery of appropriate verbal and nonverbal responses. . . . Social skills may be viewed as the coping process by which social competence is achieved. The skills – verbal and nonverbal communication, internal feelings, attitudes, and perceptions of the interpersonal context – mediate successful outcomes of social interactions that are reflected in the achievement of the individual's goals and the favorable impression made on others" (Liberman, 1988).

The way social skills are usually integrated into the process of social readjustment is figuratively illustrated by the game of tennis (Nyatanga, 1989).

> "Consider two very skilled tennis players (Becker vs Lendl). Each player has internalized the rules and the key skills of the game. Each one moves in a regular rhythm yet always anticipating and adjusting to the responses of the other. The same is necessarily applicable to the social skills. Each person must adjust eye contact, posture, proximity gestures, prosodic signals and so forth, to match or to facilitate a smooth and balanced social intercourse."

Various theoretical models have been developed in recent years about individual social skills and social competence, but the authors concerned have not been able to agree on any single theory. Morrison & Bellack (1984) favour a motor or topographical model of social skills, arguing that socially acceptable behaviour depends on successfully combining and coordinating a set of specific behavioural components which include verbal, paralingual, and non-verbal skills. People who manifest socially maladjusted behaviour either have not learnt how to implement appropriate social skills, have forgotten how to behave adaptively because of illness or long hospital residence, or are unable to implement the skills they actually possess, as a result of very strong negative feelings or affective disorders. However, social skills can also be explained and assessed by means of problem-solving models. Liberman *et al* (1985), for example, maintain that conscious, cognitive processes play a significant role in social interactions. In problem-solving models, social skills are divided into three subcomponents: social perceptual skills, i.e. the ability to interpret socially relevant stimuli correctly; the ability to solve social problems; and the ability to behave in socially acceptable and adjusted ways. Although motor elements of behaviour are important determining factors of affective behaviour, they are not thought to be as important as the cognitive processes that precede them.

Social skills training (SST)

If the number of and, above all, the quality of social skills an individual has acquired and is able to utilise are assumed to play an important role in the way a specific mental illness is defined, in the way that illness and symptoms are manifested, and in the developmental course of the illness (cf. Liberman, 1988), then social skills training must play an important part in the treatment of the chronic mentally ill. Above all, this kind of therapeutic intervention can help chronic patients attain social competence and greater personal growth, both of which are prerequisites for resocialisation. In other words, social skills training is a promising approach to reducing mental disability.

Current thinking assigns great significance to the widely recognised concept of stress/vulnerability for major psychiatric disorders. This trend also indicates how essential social skills are for fostering personal and social adjustment. The symptoms which mentally ill individuals manifest and their level of social adjustment at a particular point are seen as the result of a dynamic interplay among a number of factors. The amount of and kind of stress experienced, the individual's heightened susceptibility to stress (vulnerability), the way he or she copes with stress, and the support received from the immediate surroundings all determine how well this person will be able to function in and adapt to society.

The more individuals are able to make use of social skills, the better they will be able to deal with stress. Pharmacotherapy, however well adapted to individuals' personal needs, can help only to compensate for the long-standing vulnerability that is anchored in biochemical and neuroendocrinological abnormalities. Social interventions aim at avoiding, eliminating, or at least reducing the sources of chronic problems and tensions. Social skills training, however, is concerned with the part played actively by patients themselves in the bi-directional processes taking place between pre-existing vulnerability and manifest psychiatric illness and disability.

The first author to use the term 'social skills training' (SST) was the British psychologist Argyle (1972). Though this term was used to describe a specific method for treating interpersonal communication disorders, today's research workers employ it in a more general sense, to cover all training methods aimed at helping both emotionally well-adjusted and mentally ill individuals to behave in more acceptable and appropriate ways. Goldstein (1981) described it as "a planned, systematic teaching of behaviours needed and consciously desired by the individual in order to function in an effective and satisfactory manner over an extended period of time" (quoted by Nyatanga, 1989). Generally, social skills training aims at:

(a) changing cognitive and affective functions so as to reduce deficiences in learning and performance;

(b) eliminating inappropriate or disruptive behaviour that had itself resulted in social rejection and subjective stress;

(c) acquiring social skills which enable the individual to resume a place in social life;

(d) helping individuals to maintain environmental circumstances that encourage them to make use of acquired social skills.

The pursuit of these objectives must, however, take individuals' needs and goals as well as their strengths and social abilities into account. A programme should have the following elements:

(a) identifying behaviour and people that a patient does not feel at ease with;

(b) determining, by means of problem-solving processes, interventions which make behavioural changes possible;

(c) pinpointing environmental events that could be influenced, in order that the frequency of undesirable behaviour decreases and that of desirable behaviour increases;

(d) establishing a contract between therapist and patient in order that the desirable behaviour to be enacted is agreed on, and feedback and support given when this is actually manifested;

(e) evaluating behavioural shifts and feelings associated with certain behaviour.

With regard to the level of complexity, two main categories of skills can be distinguished in a training programme: *microsocial skills*, such as non-verbal behaviour (body contact, physical proximity and position, gestures, facial expression, eye contact), paraverbal signals (tone of voice, tone of speech, speed of speech, delivery, timing, sequencing), and verbal skills or verbal communications; and *macrosocial skills*, such as role expectations (personal hygiene, finding living accommodation, maintenance skills, work and job skills, recreational skills, etc.).

Numerous intervention techniques are regularly applied in combination with one another: modelling, demonstrating, instructing, shaping, eliminating, role-playing, rehearsing, trying out new ways of behaving, giving feed-back, giving positive reinforcement, step-by-step practice and guidance, homework assignments, generalisation training, etc. The techniques chosen depend partly on the conditions available in the institution and partly on the specific psychiatric disability that is present. These techniques are applied within the framework of different treatment settings, e.g. individual or group therapy, hospital or community-based treatment. On the whole, training methods take into account psychological learning theories, recent behavioural theories, and up-to-date educational methods. However, methods which can be deduced from the principles of human learning, especially social learning, are those most essential to SST.

Despite the large number of differing theories about social skills and of training methods, certain common denominators can be found:

(a) Interdisciplinary studies have contributed a great deal to understanding the nature of social skills in general, and the role that social skills play in chronic mental illness in particular
(b) Social skills positively correlate with social competence and mental health
(c) Learning processes are the basis of both adequate and inadequate social skills
(d) Social skills are specific for certain situations, i.e. various situations produce different skills.

In addition, three important common trends can be traced over the last decade:

(a) The central and growing importance of cognitive processes in the development of social skills
(b) Application of the same methods for both the mentally ill and the well-adjusted
(c) A shift in the priorities of diagnosis and therapy: rather than focusing on psychopathological symptoms, we give preference to diagnosing and treating deficient or disruptive behaviour and its conditions of occurrence.

General outcome

A wide range of research studies on the effectiveness of social skills training programmes for the chronic mentally ill have been conducted, mainly in the USA and Europe. From these, the following general conclusions can be drawn (cf. also Anthony & Liberman, 1986; Liberman, 1988; Roder *et al*, 1990):

(a) The severely mentally disabled are capable of acquiring new skills
(b) Skills that the mentally disabled acquire directly influence their chances of recovering
(c) The development or utilisation of environmental resources facilitates moderate-to-substantial chances of transferring trained behaviour to new situations and relationships.

These points must, however, be considered in greater detail.

Effective social skills training was first developed on the basis of numerous individual case histories and demonstration studies with small group samples.

Research studies have also been undertaken with larger clinical samples, during the last two decades. These have not only shown that chronic psychiatric patients are able to acquire and implement social skills, but also prove that appropriate training does significantly reduce the risk of relapse (Liberman, 1988; Brenner *et al*, 1990; Roder *et al*, 1990). Most of these studies examined schizophrenic patients, but Jackson *et al* (1985) recently reviewed social skills training for patients with depressive disorders.

Over the past 15 years, more than 50 such studies of psychiatric patients have been published (cf. Liberman, 1988). Brady's (1984) review indicates that social skills training is on the whole more effective than other treatment approaches in improving social behaviour and in enabling chronic patients especially to apply what they have learnt to their personal lives. If the findings reported are analysed in greater detail, the following conclusions can be drawn:

(a) Social skills training is more effective than psychotherapy with fairly handicapped patients (Matson & Senatore, 1981; Senatore *et al*, 1982)

(b) Patients with non-psychotic, unipolar depressive disorders react to social skills training better than to pharmaco- or psychotherapy (Bellack *et al*, 1981)

(c) Schizophrenic patients (Eisler *et al*, 1978), patients with social phobias (Shaw, 1979), and patients with long-term psychogenic disorders (Trower *et al*, 1978) all profited more from social skills training than from behavioural modification programmes

(d) Patients participating in day-hospital programmes can be helped more by means of social skills training than by bibliotherapy (Monti *et al*, 1982)

(e) Schizophrenic patients respond to social skills training more positively than to family therapy (Falloon *et al*, 1982)

(f) Schizophrenics can be treated more effectively by means of social skills training than by holistic therapy (Wallace *et al*, 1980; Liberman *et al*, 1980, 1981).

Robertson *et al* (1984) reviewed 16 studies pertaining to social skills training for the mentally ill. His results confirm these above-mentioned findings, and several other recent projects have also come to similar conclusions. Both Wallace & Liberman (1985) and Hogarty *et al* (1987*a*) found that after 9 and 12 months, the likelihood of relapse was significantly smaller after a treatment programme which consisted of social skills training and neuroleptic medication than after holistic therapy combined with pharmacotherapy, or after pharmacotherapy alone.

However, the question whether social skills training is really effective can hardly be answered in general. The various definitions of 'social skills' have inevitably led to differing approaches to treating such deficient or maladjusted skills. It is, therefore, extremely important for researchers to develop a differentiated approach to the assessment of therapy.

Cognitive-behavioural approaches

A major challenge for accepted social skills training results from findings that chronic psychiatric patients, particularly schizophrenics, often manifest basic attentional, perceptual, and conceptual disorders in information-processing. They show, for example, impairments of the following functions: selective attention, sustained attention, or shifting of attention; recognising, identifying, interpreting, and storing stimuli; drawing deductive and analogous conclusions; and selecting alternative ways of reacting (cf. Nuechterlein & Dawson, 1984; Brenner, 1987). These disorders in information-processing often hinder personal growth, as well as making patients incapable of acquiring new behavioural patterns or of transferring skills acquired during therapy to other situations and behaviour (generalisation). Therefore, social skills training for long-term patients must in some way take cognitive disorders into account.

Liberman *et al* (1986) took serious note of these considerations and developed a highly standardised and structured social skills training programme – '*training packages*' or '*modules*'. Basic cognitive skills are practised in these modules by utilising problem-solving abilities in relation to particular areas of skill: these include self-management of medication, symptom control, and leisure-time management. The knowledge and skills to be attained in a particular module, e.g. how to deal with medication problems, are taught by means of behavioural modification procedures (modelling by videotapes, role-playing exercises, problem-solving strategies, homework assignments, etc.). Each module consists of seven steps: steps one to four are carried out during therapy, whereas five to seven are in the patient's natural surroundings. However, an extensive series of empirical studies on the effectiveness of these modules has not yet been conducted, although first findings seem very encouraging (Liberman *et al*, 1986, 1988). Social skills training modules adapted to European conditions are currently being developed for German-speaking patients.

Bellack *et al* (1989), in assessing research up to now, were unsure whether long-term psychiatric patients can be treated more successfully by problem-solving than by motor-topographical-orientated approaches. As far as problem-solving models are concerned, currently available ones would have to be validated. In relation to the motor-orientated approach, it should be noted that most social interactions develop so quickly and so automatically that with the exception of a few standard situations, it is difficult to plan cognitive activities in advance. In other words, according to these authors, individuals' behaviour is basically evoked by social stimuli which they have perceived and processed relatively automatically. Our own clinical observations suggest that long-term psychiatric patients with a relatively low level of functioning respond quite positively to traditional behaviour modification training programmes for social skills. However, if their social skills have improved and they are capable of fulfilling more challenging social demands, they must also receive cognitive problem-solving training.

Meichenbaum & Cameron (1973) also tried to alleviate or eliminate basic attentional and conceptual disorders indirectly, by means of their self-instruction approach to therapy. This recommends that patients solve problems that demand a high level of concentration and attention by giving themselves instructions, first out loud and later silently, on how to focus their attention on a particular problem, how to continue concentrating on that same problem, and how not to let themselves be distracted. Other instructions attempt to improve skills by having patients comment on what has worked out well and encourage themselves when something has gone wrong. This procedure has, on the whole, proved to be effective, provided that a comprehensive and detailed assessment of the individual's disorders has been made before therapeutic interventions are selected (Bentall *et al*, 1987). The self-instruction approach is innovative, because it takes specific situational factors, rather than specific cognitive deficiencies, into account. This is understandable, since therapeutic self-instruction is a result of social learning theories, and not of experimental psychopathology.

A third approach to cognitive-orientated social skills training is based on information-processing models of attentional/perceptual and conceptual disorders. Both Magaro (1980) and Spaulding *et al* (1986) have reported findings from studies on training single dysfunctions through patients memorising, ignoring, or immediately reproducing information in an experimental setting. Both research teams concluded that it is possible to normalise specific cognitive disorders by means of structured and planned interventions. They also agree that skills attained on one level of functioning can be transferred to any other. Two questions, however, remain unsolved. Firstly, how far can laboratory results, attained in isolated attempts at treating individual cognitive disorders, be generalised and maintained? Secondly, is there any relationship between laboratory results and the social behaviour that is manifested in real-life situations?

Our own clinical experience with individual casework confirms this sceptical attitude (Brenner *et al*, 1980). Transferring experimental research findings on deficient functions of perceiving and processing information to actual clinical therapy is not advisable, since the abstract nature of the experimental materials and procedures hinders the transfer and utilisation of acquired skills. The social dimensions of cognitive disorders must also be taken into account explicitly. In a comprehensive model (Brenner, 1986; cf. also Spaulding *et al*, 1986), basic attentional and perceptual dysfunctions, which have an intermediate position in relation to biological abnormalities, exercise a pervasive influence on all levels of the individual's micro- and macrosocial functioning. Therefore, we have developed a therapy programme especially for the integrated treatment of cognitive, communicative, and social disorders in long-term schizophrenic patients (Brenner *et al*, 1987; Roder *et al*, 1988). In recent years, it has become known as 'the Integrated Psychological Treatment Programme' (IPT).

Various empirical studies in different centres indicate that IPT is generally an effective treatment procedure (cf. Brenner *et al*, 1990). On the other hand, more detailed research studies have shown that improved cognitive functioning does not necessarily lead to improved behavioural skills, and vice versa (Roder *et al*, 1988; cf. Mussgay & Olbrich, 1988; Hodel *et al*, 1990). This finding seems to indicate that the two skill areas are fairly independent of each other, and that the respective disorders and deficiencies do not have to be equally severe. Disorders and deficiencies in both skill areas must be individually assessed for each specific case, and only then can the appropriate treatment procedure be applied. Future research in this field will therefore have to be more deeply concerned with the following questions. Firstly, it will have to focus more on differential treatment indications. Secondly, more attention will have to be paid to which areas should be treated. Thirdly, it will have to establish an appropriate sequence of interventions, when a combination of cognitive- and behavioural-orientated strategies is implemented. In addition to this, both research findings up to now and experience with IPT in clinical work suggest that emotional processes which have a controlling effect, as well as specific characteristics of the modulation of psychophysiological activation level, must be taken into account to a greater extent (cf. Brenner, 1989).

Generalisation

Improved social behaviour acquired during therapy is not necessarily manifested in real-life situations. The problem of generalising experimentally acquired skills and knowledge was another major reason why researchers began focusing more attention on the cognitive aspects of social skills training. Until the 1970s, generalisation was not a clearly defined concept in its own right. It was considered to be a fairly passive but natural result of every change in behaviour, and was often interpreted as the logical negative outcome of stimulus–response discrimination. Nowadays, however, it is considered to be an independent goal of therapy.

Generalisation can therefore be defined as the ability to apply experimentally acquired behaviour to real-life circumstances. Scott *et al* (1983) reviewed 114 empirical studies, carried out between 1967 and 1981, on the problem of generalisation. The following results can be cited: 60% of the studies evaluated therapy (35% of them were conducted on psychiatric patients); 52% of the studies implemented only one method of evaluating generalisation, whereas 31% implemented two methods, 10% three methods, and 7% four or more methods. Only 37% of all the quoted studies assessed the length of time generalisation could be maintained (generalisation over time). Generalisation was retested on average 21 weeks later (time span ranging from 2 to 96 weeks): 85% of all the quoted studies showed positive generalisation results in one out of five dimensions (time, setting, people, role-playing scenes, and behavioural responses). On the other hand, in barely 10% of the assessed studies were psychiatric patients definitely able to transfer acquired skills and knowledge to life circumstances outside the confines of the institution. The fact that recent training programmes have been taking cognitive processes into account to a greater extent than they used to seems to have enabled patients to become more successful at generalising skills and knowledge acquired in therapy, but no extensive or detailed studies are available on this subject as yet.

Discussion

Assessing available research on competence training for the chronic mentally ill still poses various problems. Researchers often fail to give adequate information about the characteristics of the patients or the exact procedures of treatment. Above all, both the social validity of control methods and patients' ability to maintain and utilise the skills they have acquired during therapy often remain unclear. These problems must be solved before final judgement can be passed on the effectiveness of social skills training. The changes of behaviour that are measured should result in significant improvements in ensuing social life. In most studies, however, behaviour is assessed only by means of self-reports and questionnaires (pen-and-paper measures). Observing both the way patients actually behave and the way they behave in role-playing situations (even if role-playing is artificial) would be a more valid way of measuring behaviour. Since it is difficult to find alternatives, appropriate results should be backed up by measures which make it possible to draw clear conclusions on an individual's ability to adapt to real-life situations.

With regard to the question of how the effects of social skills training come about, several explanations are still open for debate, since social maladaptation can be conceptualised in different ways. First of all, both anxiety and other negative effects can make an individual unable to implement social skills in real life, and therefore unable to behave in appropriate ways. Secondly, feelings of inadequacy and self-devaluation, as well as deficiency in needed competencies, caused either by faulty learning experiences or by the loss of previously acquired skills, can also obstruct the individual's ability to manifest adjusted behaviour in real life. That is why the hypothesis of acquisition of skills that is usually made about the effects of this treatment is not, *a priori*, most plausible. On the one hand, social skills training has been proved to reduce anxiety, while, on the other, therapeutic interventions which do not utilise social skills techniques, such as group discussions about social performance which designate goals to be attained and tasks to be practised, can also result in positive behavioural changes (cf. Stravynski *et al*, 1987). Therefore, the integration of anxiety-reducing techniques and of constructive social activities could help to improve further the outcomes of social skills training.

Social skills training programmes have rarely been evaluated in terms of cost-effectiveness. Different therapy procedures and techniques demand different conditions: modelling using video play-back, for example, calls for rather costly equipment, while coaching methods call for specially experienced and qualified therapists. Cognitive-orientated training in 'experimental' settings calls for a meticulous and complicated phase of planning and diagnosis. Once this phase has been completed, training becomes less costly, because it can almost always be automatically reproduced by means of a personal computer. Cognitive-orientated group therapy, on the other hand, seems to be less costly at first glance, but this may be a false impression, because the therapists must have special training and must work with a group for longer periods of time. In addition to these observations, the amount of time necessary to attain the best possible outcome of therapy would also have to be taken into account when evaluating training programmes in terms of cost-effectiveness.

Future research should also encourage changes within the therapeutic institutions themselves, changes which enhance the generalisation, maintenance, and utilisation of trained and acquired skills outside their confines. Authors such as Hogarty *et al* (1987*b*) assert that, so far, relapses can be significantly delayed, rather than actually avoided, only as long as patients do not change to more complex life-situations or challenges. These conclusions come from having studied the way pharmacological and psychosocial therapeutic measures interact with social skills training. Deficient social skills have a particularly strong effect when the individual tries to cope with and regulate severe life stress. Advocates of social skills training claim that it may be the most important single measure for helping patients to break out of the confines of long-term hospitalisation, and resume an active role in the community. But this aspiration has up to now been only partially fulfilled.

In addition to the problems and unsolved questions that research on social competence training faces, there are also many startling incongruities between available knowledge and clinical practice. Although patients can often take part in many different social groups, they are rarely offered structured, systematic social skills training programmes, although it has been proved again and again that such programmes are particularly effective with the chronic mentally ill. Clinicians in hospitals and in other institutions need to initiate programmes that researchers have been proposing for some time.

Conclusions

Conducting social skills or competency training programmes requires the therapist to establish a new kind of relationship with the patient, as well as with society. Therapists have traditionally tended to be concerned primarily with the patient, and have been relatively neutral towards society. With social skills training, as with the newly developed psychosocial interventions, the therapist tends to try to influence both micro- and macrosocial processes – for instance, by demanding that patients have the right to participate in what is being done and said. The therapist teaches the patient to be assertive: ''Adoption of assertive behaviour . . . can assist [patients] to assume the rightful position of equality in our society'' (Smith & Kirkpatrick, 1985). Since social skills training enables individuals to assert themselves and to become active and self-reliant, without even meaning to, it is following a deep-rooted trend towards participatory democracy (the National Training Laboratory introduced democratic group processes as a means of social change; Lewin, 1943), and thus promises to be successfully utilised to a greater extent. Therapists, however, must be aware of the much higher demands that this form of therapy also makes on society, compared either with pharmacotherapy or traditional psychotherapy. As far as possible, therapists should take an objective standpoint, rather then getting involved in a 'conflict of rights'. Not enough attention has been paid to this aspect.

> ''So far not one article has appeared in the literature that speaks for the 'Rights' of those who are expected to provide food, clothing, shelter, recreation, television, and a host of other comforts . . . to those who, either by choice or incapacity, do not behave in ways acceptable to the larger community. The general thrust seems to be that the providers (or the offended) have no rights'' (Hagen, 1975).

If therapists make a constant effort to remain objective, and are competent and well qualified, they will also be able to comprehend and deal with the various defence mechanisms caused by the therapeutic measures that have been taken. If long-term psychiatric patients are to improve in social competence, their attitudes must also change. Such changes can, however, first lead to even greater problems, through the fact that they quite unexpectedly start standing up for personal rights and fighting against restrictions that had never been questioned. Also, the patient's social network has to learn to deal with this new behaviour which, although modified, is not necessarily well adjusted or completely appropriate.

The fight against major mental disorders poses very complex problems, since they can perhaps be regarded as diseases of civilisation. Whether it is chronic psychiatric illness, malnutrition, or infectious diseases that are being treated, therapy is never a process that occurs only between the therapist and the patient. All these illnesses require close and comprehensive co-operation between all structures and all members of society – universities, hospitals, health insurance companies, government, the mass media, the economy, churches, families, patients, etc.

Finally, it must not be forgotten that both the status and the role of a chronic mentally ill individual are less the result of psychiatrists' scientific points of view than of society's rejecting attitudes. The way that chronic mentally ill individuals are cared for, i.e. the service delivery system, is also less the result of the individual's specific disabilities than of prevailing socio-political and economic conditions. Such factors as public relations and financing or decision-making structures at the political and administrative level must be blamed for not allowing the chronic mentally ill to take advantage of certain therapeutic or rehabilitative services. The 'inability of integration' of certain groups of patients might actually be due to a lack of appropriate resources. 'Integration' of the chronic mentally ill must be made possible not only by teaching independent living skills, in which social competence training plays a prominent role, but also by providing in advance for the necessary socio-political and legal aspects, if the patient is to succeed in resuming a satisfying place in society.

Although social skills training is a very promising approach to treating the chronic mentally ill, it must be planned with prevailing conditions and goals kept in mind. It must be an integral part of a comprehensive treatment or rehabilitation process which takes various therapeutic measures into account, and must go hand in hand with measures aimed at influencing the patient's social environment. These measures can range from therapeutic interventions directed at the patient's closest social relationships to far-reaching socio-political measures. Only this combination can result in effective social skills training. However, programmes for improving social competence should be implemented more often than they are at present, even in situations where this is not yet possible on a full-scale basis. Every time a programme is implemented, new insights can be gained. Working with the chronic mentally ill should always remind us that suffering can never be completely overcome, and that illness can never be totally eradicated. Therefore, no matter how problematic the battle against suffering and illness might be, it is always worth the greatest possible efforts by all concerned.

References

ANTHONY, W. A. & LIBERMAN, R. P. (1986) The practice of psychiatric rehabilitation: historical, conceptual, and research base. *Schizophrenia Bulletin*, **12**, 542–559.

—— HOWELL, J. & DANLEY, K. (1984) The vocational rehabilitation of the psychiatrically disabled. In *The Chronically Mentally Ill: Research and Services* (ed. M. Mirabi), pp. 215–237. New York: SP Books.

ARGYLE, M. (1972) *The Psychology of Interpersonal Behaviour.* Harmondsworth: Penguin.

BELLACK, A. S., HERSEN, M. & HIMMELHOCH, J. M. (1981) Social skills training compared with pharmacotherapy and psychotherapy in the treatment of unipolar depression. *American Journal of Psychiatry,* **138,** 1562–1567.

——, TURNER, S. M., HERSEN, M., *et al* (1984) An examination of the efficacy of social skills training for chronic schizophrenic patients. *Hospital and Community Psychiatry,* **35,** 1023–1028.

——, MORRISON, R. L. & MUESER, K. T. (1989) Social problem solving in schizophrenia. *Schizophrenia Bulletin,* **15,** 101–116.

BENTALL, R., HIGSON, P. & LOWE, C. (1987) Teaching self-instructions to chronic schizophrenic patients: efficacy and generalisation. *Behavioral Psychotherapy,* **15,** 58–76.

BRADY, J. P. (1984) Social skills training for psychiatric patients. II: Clinical outcome studies. *American Journal of Psychiatry,* **141,** 491–493.

BRENNER, H. D. (1987) On the importance of cognitive disorders in treatment and rehabilitation. In *Psychosocial Treatment of Schizophrenia,* (eds. J. S. Strauss, W. Böker & H. D. Brenner). Lewiston, NY: Huber.

—— (1989) The treatment of basic psychological dysfunctions from a systemic point of view. *British Journal of Psychiatry,* **155,** 74–83.

——, STRAMKE, W. G., MEWES, J., *et al* (1980) A treatment program, based on training of cognitive and communicative functions, in the rehabilitation of chronic schizophrenic patients. *Nervenarzt,* **51,** 106–112.

——, HODEL, B., KUBE, G., *et al* (1987) Cognitive therapy with schizophrenics: analysis of the problem and experimental results. *Nervenarzt,* **58,** 72–83.

——, KRAEMER, S., HERMANUTZ, M., *et al* (1990) Cognitive treatment in schizophrenia: models and interventions. In *Schizophrenia: Concepts, Vulnerability and Intervention,* (eds. E. R. Straube & K. Hahlweg), pp. 161–191. Berlin: Springer.

EISLER, R. M., BLANCHARD, E. B. & FITTS, H. (1978) Social skill training with and without modelling for schizophrenic and non-psychotic hospitalized psychiatric patients. *Behavior Modification,* **2,** 147–172.

FALLOON, I. R. H. & TALBOT, R. E. (1981) Persistent auditory hallucinations: coping mechanisms and implications for management. *Psychological Medicine,* **11,** 329–339.

——, BOYD, J. L., McGILL, C. W., *et al* (1982) Family management in the prevention of schizophrenia. *New England Journal of Medicine,* **306,** 1437–1440.

FREY, W. D. (1984) Functional assessment in the '80s: a conceptual enigma, a technical challenge. In *Functional Assessment in Rehabilitation,* (eds A. Halpern & M. Fuhrer). New York: Brooke.

GOLDSTEIN, A. P. (1981) *Psychosocial Skills Training: The Structured Learning Technique.* Oxford: Pergamon.

GOLDSTROM, I. & MANDERSCHEID, R. (1982) The chronically mentally ill: a descriptive analysis from the uniform client data instrument. *Community Support Services Journal,* **2,** 4–9.

GRUENBERG, E. M. (1969) From practice to theory: community mental-health services and the nature of psychoses. *Lancet, i,* 721–724.

HAGEN, R. L. (1975) Behavioral therapies and the treatment of schizophrenics. *Schizophrenia Bulletin,* **13,** 70–96.

HARROW, M., GRINKER, P. R., SILVERSTEIN, M. L., *et al* (1978) Is modern-day schizophrenic outcome still negative? *American Journal of Psychiatry,* **135,** 1156–1162.

HODEL, B., BRENNER, H. D. & MERLO, M. (1990) Cognitive and social training for chronic schizophrenic patients: a comparison between two types of therapeutic interventions. In *Psychiatry: a World Perspective,* vol. 3 (ed. C. N. Stefanis), pp. 768–773, (International Congress Series 900–3). Amsterdam: Elsevier.

HOGARTY, G. E. & ANDERSON, C. M. (1987a) A controlled study of family therapy, social skills training and maintenance chemotherapy in the aftercare treatment of schizophrenic patients: preliminary effects on relapse and expressed emotion at one year. In *Psychosocial*

Treatment of Schizophrenia (eds J. S. Strauss, W. Böhr & H. D. Brenner). Lewiston, NY: Huber.

———, ——— & REISS, D. J. (1987*b*) Family psychoeducation, social skills training, and medication in schizophrenia: the long and short of it. *Psychopharmacology Bulletin*, **23**, 12–13.

JACKSON, H. J., MOSS, J. D. & SOLINSKI, S. (1985) Social skills training: an effective treatment for unipolar non-psychotic depression? *Australian and New Zealand Journal of Psychiatry*, **19**, 342–353.

LÉVI-STRAUSS, C. (1945) L'Analyse structurale en linguistique et en anthropologie. *World Journal of the Linguistic Circle of New York*, **2**, 1–21.

LEWIN, K. (1943) Forces behind food habits and methods of change. *Bulletin of National Research Council*, **108**, 35–65.

LIBERMAN, R. P. (1982) Social factors in schizophrenia. In *Annual Review of the American Psychiatric Association*, (vol. 1), (ed L. Grinspoon). Washington, DC: American Psychiatric Press.

——— (ed.) (1988) Psychiatric Rehabilitation of Chronic Mental Patients. New York: American Psychiatric Press.

———, WALLACE, C. J., VAUGHN, C. E., *et al* (1980) Social and family factors in the course of schizophrenia: Toward an interpersonal problem-solving therapy for schizophrenics and their relatives. In *Psychotherapy of Schizophrenia: Current Status and New Directions*, (eds J. Strauss, S. Fleck, M. B. Bowers, Jr, *et al*), pp. 21–54. New York: Plenum.

———, ———, FALLOON, I. R. H., *et al* (1981) Interpersonal problem-solving therapy for schizophrenics and their families. *Comprehensive Psychiatry*, **22**, 627–629.

———, MASSELL, H. K., MOSK, M., *et al* (1985) Social skills training for chronic mental patients. *Hospital and Community Psychiatry*, **36**, 396–403.

———, MUESER, K. T. & WALLACE, C. J. (1986) Social skills training for schizophrenic individuals at risk for relapse. *American Journal of Psychiatry*, **143**, 523–526.

LINN, M. W., KLETT, C. J. & CAFFEY, E. M. (1980) Foster home characteristics and psychiatric patient outcome. *Archives of General Psychiatry*, **41**, 157–161.

MAGARO, P. A. (1980) Cognition in Schizophrenia and Paranoia. The Integration of Cognitive Processes. Hillsdale, NY: L. Erlbaum Assocation.

MATSON, J. L. & SENATORE, V. A. (1981) A comparison of traditional psychotherapy and social skills training for improving interpersonal functioning of mentally retarded adults. *Behavioral Therapy*, **12**, 369–382.

MEICHENBAUM, D. & CAMERON, R. (1973) Training schizophrenics to talk to themselves: a means of developing attentional controls. *Behavioral Therapy*, **4**, 515–534.

MONTI, P. M., CORRIVEAU, D. P. & CURRAN, J. P. (1982) Social skills training for psychiatric patients: treatment and outcome. In *Social Skills Training: A Practical Handbook for Assessment and Treatment*, (eds J. P. Curran & P. M. Monti). New York: Guilford.

MORRISON, R. L. & BELLACK, A. S. (1984) Social skills training. In *Schizophrenia: Treatment, Management and Rehabilitation*, (ed. A. S. Bellack), pp. 247–279. Orlando, FL: Grune & Stratton.

MUSSGAY, L. & OLBRICH, R. (1988) Trainingsprogramme in der Behandlung kotnitiver Defizite Schizophrener: Eine kritische Würdigung. *Klinische Psychologie*, **12**(4), 341–353.

NUECHTERLEIN, K. & DAWSON, M. A. (1984) Heuristic vulnerability/stress model of schizophrenic episodes. *Schizophrenia Bulletin*, **10**, 300–312.

NYATANGA, L. (1989) Social skills training: some ideas on its origin, nature and application. *Nurse Education Today*, **9**, 56–63.

O'MALLEY, J. W. (1977) Research perspective on social competence. *Merrill-Palmer Quarterly*, **23**, 29–44.

ROBERTSON, I., RICHARDSON, M. & YOUNGSON, S. (1984) Social skills training with mentally handicapped people: a review. *British Journal of Clinical Psychology*, **23**, 241–264.

RODER, V. (1988) Untersuchungen zur Effektivität kognitiver Therapieinterventionen mit schizophrenen Patienten. Dissertation phil.hist. Fakultät, Universität Bern.

———, BRENNER, H. D., KIENZLE, N., *et al* (1988) *Integriertes Psychologisches Therapieprogramm für schizophrene Patienten (IPT)*. München, Weinheim: Psychologie Verlags Union.

——, ECKMAN, T. A., BRENNER, H. D., *et al* (1990) Behavior therapy of schizophrenic patients. In *Handbook of Schizophrenia. vol. 5. Psychosocial Treatment of Schizophrenia*, (ed. M. I. Herz), pp. 107–134. Amsterdam: Elsevier.

SCOTT, R. R., HIMADI, W. & KEANE, T. M. (1983) A review of generalization in social skills training: suggestions for future research. In *Progress in Behavior Modification*, (eds M. Hersen, R. M. Eisler & P. M. Miller). New York: Academic Press.

SENATORE, V., MATSON, J. L. & KAZDIN, A. E. (1982) A comparison of behavioral methods to train social skills to mentally retarded adults. *Behavioral Therapy*, **13**, 313–324.

SHADISH, W. R., JR & BOOTZIN, R. R. (1984) The social integration of psychiatric patients in nursing homes. *American Journal of Psychiatry*, **141**, 1203–1207.

SHAW, P. (1979) A comparison of three behaviour therapies in the treatment of social phobia. *British Journal of Psychiatry*, **134**, 620–623.

SMITH, S. L. & KIRKPATRICK, M. (1985) Changing attitudes of disabled females through assertiveness training. *Rehabilitation Nursing*, **10**, 19–21.

SPAULDING, W. D., STORMS, L., GOODRICH, V., *et al* (1986) Applications of experimental psychopathology in psychiatric rehabilitation. *Schizophrenia Bulletin*, **12**, 560–577.

STRAVYNSKI, A., GREY, S. & ELIE, R. (1987) Outline of the therapeutic process in social skills training with socially dysfunctional patients. *Journal of Consulting and Clinical Psychology*, **55**, 224–228.

SYLPH, J. A., ROSS, H. E. & KEDWARD, H. B. (1978) Social disability in chronic psychiatric patients. *American Journal of Psychiatry*, **134**, 1391–1394.

TROWER, P., BRYANT, B. & ARGYLE, M. (1978) *Social Skills and Mental Health*. London: Methuen.

WALLACE, C. J., NELSON, C. J., LIBERMAN, R. P., *et al* (1980) A review and critique of social skills training with schizophrenic patients. *Schizophrenia Bulletin*, **6**, 42–63.

—— & LIBERMAN, R. P. (1985) Social skills training for patients with schizophrenia: a controlled clinical trial. *Psychiatry Research*, **15**, 239–247.

9 Integrating mental health in primary health care

DAVID GOLDBERG

It will be argued here that an important component of a future community-based psychiatric service should be collaborative work between specialised members of the mental health team and general practitioners. Much of this work should take place in primary care settings, but the greatest threat to future services is a fragmentation of responsibility among the members of what were once called 'multidisciplinary teams'.

However, these are minority views. It is salutary to recall that a full-scale conference held in London in 1986 between the Department of Health and the Royal College of Psychiatrists to discuss the future of the UK mental health services contained no mention of psychiatrists (or, indeed, anyone else) working in primary care settings, and the description of the future "ideal service", in the book resulting from that conference, considers only those who have ever been admitted to an in-patient bed (Wilkinson & Freeman, 1986, pp. 49–56).

The importance of primary care

The World Health Organization has recently completed a study of the referral pathways followed by patients coming into mental health care for the first time in 11 widely different countries (Gater *et al*, 1990). In all the European countries involved (Czechoslovakia, the UK, Portugal, and Spain) and in both Cuba and Yemen, between 63% and 81% of all new cases seen were referred by general practitioners; even in developing countries, where direct referrals from the community and referrals from native healers were more common, between a quarter and one-third of patients were so referred. In all countries except Indonesia, referral to a mental health professional emerged as a predominantly medical matter, so that the training of staff in these settings to recognise and manage psychological disorders becomes a matter of some concern to mental health professionals.

115

In developing countries, the WHO has in recent years been attempting to incorporate mental health services into primary care. Medical officers and multipurpose care workers are trained both to recognise and to treat targeted psychiatric disorders, often using simple diagnostic algorithms. The psychiatrists play a part in providing training to primary care staff, and may themselves come to carry out a weekly or monthly clinic, to see patients who have caused difficulty for the clinic staff. In these countries, primary care medical clinics have therefore become an integral part of the psychiatric services.

In Europe, psychiatric services are largely independent of primary care: mental health professionals work either in hospital out-patient settings, in purpose-built community mental health centres (CMHCs), or in private practice. However, there have been recent developments in the UK and Portugal to coordinate care, and psychiatrists are working closely with primary care doctors in the Netherlands and Italy. In the Netherlands, Gersons (1990) has argued that the relationship between general practitioners on the one hand, and mental health professionals working in CMHCs, on the other is inherently competitive: the general practitioner (GP) "must constantly defend his territory against the specialist mental health services". General practitioners are said "not to enjoy" relinquishing patients to a psychiatrist, and the supposed stigma of mental illness is used as a fig-leaf to hide this reluctance. Neither the GPs themselves nor the Dutch general public is said to wish to change this *status quo*. It seems likely that the situation described by Gersons applies to those health care systems where both primary care doctor and mental health professional are working on a fee-for-service basis, and that collaborative patterns of working are favoured by health care systems where medical care is free at the point of delivery of service.

However, even in the UK, a movement of psychiatrists into primary care clinics is a relatively recent phenomenon, despite the fact that the National Health Service has been running for just over 40 years. In 1975, Brook & Cooper could write that, "most psychiatrists in their NHS work see little of the local general practitioner", although they admitted that "information is lacking about numbers of professional workers already operating in community teams, and their distribution across the country". In their review of patterns of relationship between general practitioner and psychiatrist, these authors could do little more than stress the importance of the field, and to review fewer than a dozen scattered accounts of various examples of service that had been written up at the time (e.g. Brook *et al*, 1966). Writing in a similar vein, Tyrer (1984) observed that the only regular 'liaison' achieved by most of his colleagues was with hospital doctors, and that their only service in the community was the domiciliary visit. Despite these criticisms, increasing numbers of consultant psychiatrists were deciding to move into primary care settings throughout the 1970s.

Psychiatrists in primary care settings

Strathdee & Williams (1984) carried out a postal survey of all psychiatrists in England & Wales, and were able to establish that clinics in general practice began to become much more numerous from 1970 onwards, so that by the time of their survey, about 20% of psychiatrists were spending at least one session per week in primary care settings. The ones carrying out such work tended to be younger than their non-involved colleagues. Two-thirds did these clinics in addition to their other commitments, and only 33% instead of previous out-patient commitments.

Similar developments have been occurring in Scotland. Pullen & Yellowlees (1988) showed that, by 1985, no fewer than 56% of Scottish psychiatrists were working in primary care settings. The advantages mentioned of the new pattern of working were better compliance and better information about patients from GPs, as well as mutual education and learning. The disadvantages were longer travel time, time wasted when patients defaulted, poor accommodation, and no secretarial support. In some regions all psychiatrists were working in primary care, while the lowest rate – 33% – was in Glasgow. More than 85% of those working in primary care see new referrals, conduct short-term treatment, and give long-term treatment and support in these settings.

The system whereby in-patient services form the centre-piece of mental illness services, but where there are peripheral units in areas of greater morbidity has been described as the 'hive system' by Tyrer (1985). These peripheral units "may be day hospitals, community clinics or mental health centres, but not new large in-patient units". Such community clinics may be in community mental health centres or in primary care. They are said to lead to greater referral rates, to earlier detection of psychiatric illness, and to the prevention of relapse among patients who show poor compliance. These are bold claims, for which there is as yet only partial evidence. In an earlier paper, Tyrer (1984) described psychiatric clinics in general practice. Clinics were held at intervals of from one week to one month, depending on the size of population served: despite a reduction in hospital out-patient clinics, there was a net increase of 1.5 clinics/week for the participating psychiatrist.

It remains to ask why there has been such a large-scale movement into the community by the UK's consultant psychiatrists, and by increasing numbers of their trainees. Part of the explanation must be sought in the run-down of the mental hospitals, and the failure of health authorities to provide purpose-built accommodation for mental health staff in the community. Williams & Balestrieri (1989) have argued that regions with the greatest number of such clinics are those where there has been the greatest reduction in annual admission rates for mental illnesses. This is undoubtedly so, but the direction of the causal relationship is less clear than the authors suggest.

Patterns of collaboration

An early paper by Williams & Clare (1981) described three sorts of relationship which might occur between visiting psychiatrists and their hosts in primary care. These were the "replacement model", where the psychiatrist replaces GP as doctor of first contact; the "increased throughput model", where GPs were encouraged to refer more patients; and the "liaison-attachment" model, where the role of the psychiatrist is to strengthen GPs in their therapeutic role.

In practice, only a minority of the consultants who later answered the questionnaire were found to correspond to this theoretical classification. The largest group – almost two-thirds of those who replied – were found to be operating a *shifted out-patient model*. Here, the psychiatrist carries out what is in effect a usual out-patient session, but it happens to be held in a primary care clinic, rather than within the walls of the hospital. The psychiatrist undertakes both assessment and treatment. The next biggest group (28%) operate a *consultation model*: here, the psychiatrist gives assistance to GPs by assessing patients and discussing management with the referring doctor, who is to be responsible for treatment. Some psychotherapists who operate this model may not see patients at all, but give Balint-type seminars, and aim to change the attitudes and modify the therapeutic skills of the GP concerned. The smallest group – only 5% – was the *liaison attachment model*, where the psychiatrist institutes working and training links with other disciplines – social workers, community psychiatric nurses, health visitors, and psychologists. Here the psychiatrist has a largely supervisory and training role, and may not see patients at all.

Generally speaking, both the psychiatrists and their hosts in general practice were enthusiastic about the new service. Among the other advantages mentioned are providing support for the primary care team, and providing educational functions by seminars, lectures, and case-conferences.

We have recently conducted a medical audit of the primary care clinics held by consultant psychiatrists working in central Manchester. All nine of the consultants carry out such clinics: six of them (together with two trainees) carry out 'shifted out-patient' clinics, and three now undertake what they have described as 'consultation-liaison' clinics (Creed & Marks, 1989). The latter type of attachment is closest to Strathdee & Williams' (1984) 'consultation' model: it consists of the psychiatrist attending the primary care team meeting and discussing the management of several problem patients who are mentioned there. After the meeting, there may be one or two patients booked to be seen. Where possible, these are seen together with the GP, and it is clear to the patient that the GP will continue to be in charge of treatment. If it is not possible for the GP to stay and see the patient, the psychiatrist will discuss the patient directly with the doctor, as well as write a letter, and will usually arrange for the GP to continue to be responsible for treatment. At the end of a given session in a primary care clinic, our consultants completed a form giving details of which staff they had seen, how many patients and relatives had been seen, and the diagnoses of those patients. Our preliminary data are concerned with 58 sessions carried out using the 'shifted out-patient' model, and 26 sessions using the 'consultation liaison model'.

During the first group of sessions, consultants saw on average 5.3 patients and discussed between three and four more with community nurses seen then. However, of the total of 308 patients seen, only 14 (4.5%) were new patients, the others being old patients seen for follow-up. Furthermore, although the clinics were being held in primary care clinics, contact between the psychiatrists and the GPs was very slight, and frequently non-existent: less than 1% of time was spent in this way, and not a single message had been left by a GP for the visiting psychiatrist in any of the 58 clinics included in the audit. In contrast, those using the 'consultation-liaison model' directly saw, on average, only 1.8 patients per session, but of 42 patients seen, 19 (45%) were new. In addition to those seen directly, a further four to six other patients were discussed during each session with the GPs: therefore, the total number of patients seen directly or discussed was about the same in each model. However, in this second model, psychiatrists spent between 30% and 100% of their time with the GPs, so that there was far more opportunity to influence events in the primary care setting.

The diagnostic breakdown of the patients seen in each setting is also quite instructive, as shown in Table 9.1.

It is disturbing that whichever model is used, patients with chronic brain syndrome, drug dependence, or mental handicap are not being seen: yet all these patients are seen by a hospital-based service. Of course, with greater numbers, some of these patients are bound to make an appearance: but it seems unlikely that very many will be seen unless steps are taken to alter the models of service offered. The shifted out-patient model seems to be offering a fairly conventional out-patient service for patients with functional psychoses, while the alternative model is clearly dealing with a much wider range of morbidity.

Creed & Marks (1989) have explained how the 'consultation-liaison' model effectively reaches a much wider set of patients. Where major illnesses are concerned, in addition to those patients who are prepared to see the psychiatrist, advice is available on the substantial group of psychotic patients who prefer not to be seen by the psychiatrist. Where common, minor illness is concerned, the psychiatrist of course sees only a small proportion of those that exist in the clinic population, but the GP gains advice about many patients who have been seen but are not referred.

It should be stressed that many of these findings came as a surprise to the psychiatrists who very kindly completed the survey forms. This is one of the achievements of a fairly simple audit procedure. It is clear that both

TABLE 9.1
Diagnostic breakdown of patients seen in different settings

Diagnostic group	Shifted out-patient	Consultation-liaison
Anxiety states	0.6%	12.0%
Anxiety/depression	7.5%	35.7%
Bipolar illness	24.6%	14.2%
Schizophrenia	62.3%	16.7%
Chronic brain syndrome	1.0%	0.0%
Drug dependence	0.0%	7.1%
Alcoholic dependence	0.33%	2.4%
Mental handicap	0.66%	0.0%
Other	1.6%	11.9%
Number	308	42

models need some attention if psychiatrists are to continue to see new patients, if psychotherapy is to continue to be offered, and if patients with 'unattractive' disorders are to be offered a service. It is noteworthy that Tyrer's figures also suggested that the number of new patients seen was actually reduced in the clinics organised in primary care, and that he found himself seeing many 'graduates' of the psychiatric service: this is reminiscent of the 'shifted out-patient' model described here, which is the commonest type of clinic offered throughout the UK. If such clinics are indeed to offer an acceptable alternative to the old hospital-based service, it seems clear that much work remains to be done in changing not only the attitudes of GPs, but also those of the psychiatrists themselves.

Community psychiatric nurses

In their review of the relationship between the primary care team and the mental health service, Brook & Cooper (1975) described the work of the community psychiatric nurse (CPN) (as it then was) in the following terms:

"The emphasis is placed firmly on major mental illness . . . the community nurse pays visits to ensure that drugs are being taken as prescribed; to give injections of long-acting phenothiazines; to check for signs of mental deterioration; to supervise patients' general welfare and to provide support for the relatives."

Times have changed. In many parts of the country, CPNs have cut themselves loose from the multidisciplinary team, and offer their own independent service directly to GPs. Wooff *et al* (1986) used case register data to compare the clinical work done by CPNs and psychiatrists: these CPNs still accepted referrals from both sources. It was shown that although psychiatrists referred predominantly schizophrenic and demented patients to the CPNs, the GPs referred depressed and anxious patients, thus the overall diagnostic case mix for the CPNs was the same as that for the psychiatrists. It was also shown that the increased numbers of CPNs employed by the health authority in the period under review had not had the effect of decreasing the strain on the remainder of the psychiatric service. Indeed, if anything, the rest of the service were seeing even more patients than before, so that the effect of the CPNs was to make treatment available to a wider range of patients with minor disorders (20% of CPN patients were not seen by anyone else). Nor could it be shown that increases in the CPN service caused a reduction in the rate of accumulation of new long-stay patients.

In a further, more detailed observational study, Wooff *et al* (1988) showed that CPNs spent significantly less time with psychotic patients than they did with patients suffering from neuroses, and that they had fewer contacts with other professionals than did mental health social workers. Finally, Wooff & Goldberg (1988) found that CPNs had increasing case-loads, with little supervision from their professional managers and in relative isolation from other members of the mental health team.

The importance of teamwork was stressed in the government White Paper *Better Services for the Mentally Ill* (1975), and was reiterated in the *Report on a Study of Communtiy Care* (DHSS, 1981). Wooff & Goldberg stress the danger of patients with long-term needs being offered an 'acute' service model, with long-term provision being limited to the maintenance of medication. Such a model of service will ensure that the worst characteristics of life in the 'back wards' of mental hospitals will be perpetuated in the era of 'community care'.

Clinical psychologists in primary care settings

There has been a large expansion in the numbers of clinical psychologists in the UK in recent years, but following the Trethowan Report they have split away from clinical psychiatry, and an increasing number identify their main interest in non-psychiatric specialties. By 1985, there were 1734 posts for clinical psychologists, as compared with 1186 consultant psychiatrists in general psychiatry, and 677 in various specialties. In many centres, clinical psychology – far from working in a collaborative way with other mental health professions – appears to be establishing a service parallel to psychiatry, with direct referrals and its own waiting lists.

Many clinical psychologists now undertake sessions in primary care, where they accept direct referrals from the general practitioners, in much the same way as psychiatrists who carry out similar clinics. In many ways, these developments are excellent, and provide a service which is appreciated by patients and by the referring GPs. However, there is a problem. The movement of clinical psychologists away from collaborative work with psychiatrists has meant that there are now many fewer to deal with problems posed by the more severely ill. It is not that the patients seen by them in primary care do not merit care, but merely that they represent common, minor problems, compared with the less frequent, more severe problems seen in psychiatric units. Brandon (unpublished) has pointed out that the competitiveness which is developing between psychology and the rest of the mental health service is destructive both to the best interests of the patients and the most appropriate use of resources.

Effects of the new services on admission rates

Tyrer *et al* (1984) showed that practices in Nottingham which had psychiatrists attached to them produced a greater reduction in admissions than those which did not: whereas the former reduced admissions from 225 to 179/1000, the latter reduced theirs only from 189 to 170/1000. However, the detached observer will note that the index group was starting with a very much higher rate of admissions than the control group, and that even at the end of the observation period, the controls were admitting fewer patients than the index group. Thus, these findings are really not at all conclusive – they may just illustrate a 'ceiling effect'. Furthermore, the index practices were seeing fewer new referrals than the control practices: their increased work load was accounted for by a great increase in 'old referrals'. The service described by these authors seems to ensure that patients who had once been known to the psychiatric services become known to them again, and this may indeed have preventive value.

McKechnie *et al* (1981) found fewer admissions in practices served by a specialised psychiatric team than in those not so served. In a similar vein, de Girolamo *et al* (1988) compared two contrasting services in Italy. The "hospital-orientated" service in Cremona had only 0.1 beds per 1000 at risk, no community facilities, and only a single community nurse, while the "well-developed community services" in Mantua had a mere 0.06 beds/1000, but made up for it with 20 CPNs, three community mental health centres, and four out-patient clinics. The authors show that the former service was associated with an annual admission rate of 3.57/1000, while the latter had only 1.57/1000. They conclude that this is a good thing. However, both these rates are so far below the rates one would expect in a well-resourced service that one could argue that one form of privation was being compared with another.

More recently, Williams & Balestrieri (1989) show that those regions of England which have developed psychiatric clinics in general practice are also those with the steepest decrease in psychiatric admissions. However, the direction of the causal link is not so easy to discern: were the psychiatrists lured out into the community, or were they driven there?

The fragmentation of services

In the UK, the decision to move into primary care has been made by each profession alone, without reference to the others. Thus, psychiatrists, clinical psychologists, and community nurses have each offered separate services in primary care settings, and general practitioners have been pleased to accommodate them. Health administrators have been pleased to allow these developments, since the marginal cost to the Health Authorities in terms of capital and recurrent revenue is very low. There are still many examples of community psychiatric teams offering a range of skills depending upon the patient's need, but this is no longer the prevalent model. No central leadership comes from the Department of Health, and each national professional body speaks mainly for the interests of its members.

The consequences of what is happening are serious, and do not appear to have been examined in any systematic way. It seems certain that the types of patient now offered help are different from those offered help formerly. A practice with an attached clinical psychologist may, for example, be able to offer help to agoraphobic housewives and to the many patients with anxiety-related symptoms who would not previously have received care at all. This is a good thing, but it is a good that deserves to be weighed against the patients who are *not* now receiving a high-quality service. These include those with chronic psychotic illnesses, those with various degrees of brain damage, and many with moderate and severe mental handicap. It is also important that patients receive interventions that are determined by their needs, rather than the therapeutic strategies that happen to be favoured by the mental health professional attached to a particular clinic.

Only a coordinated, multidisciplinary team, which can refer patients to its members for specialised advice or intervention, and which has a manager who is responsible for ensuring that there is a proper distribution of resources among the various competing needs of the population at risk, can achieve these ends. The problems that prevent such a state of affairs from coming about are by no means insurmountable, but they show little sign of being surmounted. We are up against competing claims for professional hegemony, and we are not helped by a government whose philosophy encourages each profession to sell itself on the market.

Envoi

The forces that have driven psychiatrists into primary care settings in the UK are inexorable: they will not go away. However, it remains to ask whether an extramural service can be wholly based in this setting. There are good reasons for supposing that it cannot. In the first place, it is difficult to offer a comprehensive service in this setting. There is always an additional need for day-care facilities and rehabilitation facilities which cannot be added on to primary care. Secondly, there is the simple logistics of the operation: there are not enough psychiatrists or clinical psychologists to allow clinics to be held in every general practice throughout the UK. It seems likely that such services will continue to be offered in larger group practices, because they have advantages which cannot be denied: many patients prefer them; there is better compliance with treatment, and more opportunity to advise GPs about a wide range of patients with psychological problems.

However, for patients attending single-handed GPs, and even for some who attend large group practices, there will continue to be a need for a community-based, co-ordinated psychiatric service, offering a range of facilities that cannot readily be assimilated into a primary care framework. These facilities can either be hospital based, or they can be in peripheral community mental health centres; but they will be necessary. Describing the optimal managerial structure for such teams, and specifying the kinds of desirable buildings that will be needed in the community, in addition to facilities in primary care, are important tasks for the coming decade.

References

BROOK, A., BLEASDALE, J. K., DOWLING, ST. J., *et al* (1966) *Journal of the Royal College of General Practitioners*, **11**, 184–194.

BROOK, P. & COOPER, B. (1975) Community mental health care: primary team and specialist services. *Journal of the Royal College of General Practitioners*, **25**, 93–110.

CREED, F. & MARKS, B. (1989) Liaison psychiatry in general practice. *Journal of the Royal College of General Practitioners*, **39**, 514–517.

DE GIROLAMO, G., MORS, O., ROSSI, G., *et al* (1988) Admission to general hospital psychiatric wards in Italy. 1. A comparison of two catchment areas with differing provision of out-patient care. *International Journal of Social Psychiatry*, **34**, 248–257.

GATER, R., SOUSA, B. de A., CARAVEO, J., *et al* (1991) The pathways to psychiatric care: a cross-cultural study. *Psychological Medicine* (in press).

GERSONS, B. P. R. (1990) The competitive relationship between mental health services and family practice. In *The Public Health Impact of Mental Disorder*, (eds D. Goldberg & D. Tantam), pp. 214–220. Basel: Hans Huber.

MCKECHNIE, A. A., PHILIP, A. E. & RAMAGE, J. G. (1981) Psychiatric services in primary care: specialised or not? *Journal of the Royal College of General Practitioners*, **31**, 611–614.

PULLEN, I. M. & YELLOWLEES, A. (1988) Scottish psychiatrists in primary care settings: a silent majority. *British Journal of Psychiatry*, **153**, 663–666.

STRATHDEE, G. & WILLIAMS, P. (1984) A survey of psychiatrists in primary care: the silent growth of a new service. *Journal of the Royal College of General Practitioners*, **34**, 615–618.

TYRER, P. (1984) Psychiatric clinics in general practice. *British Journal of Psychiatry*, **145**, 9–14.

—— (1985) The hive system. a model for a psychiatric service. *British Journal of Psychiatry*, **146**, 571–575.

——, SIEVEWRIGHT, N. & WOLLERTON, S. (1984) General practice psychiatric clinics: impact on psychiatric service. *British Journal of Psychiatry*, **145**, 15–19.

WILLIAMS, P. & CLARE, A. (1981) Changing patterns of psychiatric care. *British Medical Journal*, **232**, 375–377.

—— & BALESTRIERI, M. (1989) Psychiatric clinics in general practice: do they reduce admissions? *British Journal of Psychiatry*, **154**, 67–71.
WILKINSON, G. & FREEMAN, H. (1986) *The Provision of Mental Health Services in Britain: The Way Ahead*. London: Gaskell.
WOOFF, K., GOLDBERG, D. P. & FRYERS, T. (1986) Patients in receipt of community psychiatric nursing care in Salford, 1976–82. *Psychological Medicine*, **16**, 407–414.
——, —— & —— (1988) The practice of community psychiatric nursing and mental health social work in Salford: some implications for community care. *British Journal of Psychiatry*, **152**, 783–798.
—— & —— (1988) Further observations on the practice of community care in Salford: differences between community psychiatric nursing and mental health social workers. *British Journal of Psychiatry*, **153**, 30–37.

Discussion: TOM FAHY

Professor Goldberg argues that there should be a high priority for on-site integration of primary with psychiatric care in any future mental health service. Curiously, he does not state the evidential basis for this position: rather, he assumes that it is evident from the allegedly irreversible drift of younger UK psychiatrists into GP liaison work over the last 15 years. He sketches this trend with admirable objectivity, but in so doing, effectively dismantles his own thesis. Thus, he notes with dismay the disintegration of the multidisciplinary psychiatric team and the adverse consequences which flow from this. He astutely observes that an apparent correlation between run-down of beds and GP liaison activity does not necessarily imply the direction of any causal relationship (''were they [psychiatrists] lured out or driven out?'').

The paper is written almost exclusively from a UK standpoint. The organisation of the NHS strongly favours psychiatrist–GP liaison, as Goldberg is at pains to point out, but in other EC Member States, conditions may not be so favourable. In Ireland, for example, where a high bed-to-population ratio persists, the bulk of a GP's income derives from private practice. No incentive is offered to psychiatrists to engage in domiciliary work, and GPs are not rewarded for working part-time in mental health services. Large group practices of the UK type have been slow to appear. Such circumstances do not encourage GPs to spend their valuable time in conference with psychiatrists. Not surprisingly, there has been no drift of Irish psychiatrists, comparable to that which has taken place in the UK towards primary care. In Ireland, however, the psychiatric multidisciplinary team remains intact, and the activities (and loyalties) of Irish CPNs, psychologists, and social workers still resemble those in the UK in the 1970s. It might be thought from this that the attitudes of Irish GPs differ from those of their UK colleagues with respect to their psychiatric patients, but this is not the case, as an Irish national survey showed some 15 years ago. It emerged from this survey that GPs who were younger and in urban private practice had more sophisticated 'psychological' approaches to psychiatric cases than had their older, rural colleagues with little private practice. This confirms that medical attitudes in the 'soft' area of psychiatry are shaped primarily by socio-economic conditions of medical practice.

This paper acknowledges the formidable attitudinal and administrative barriers to effective GP–psychiatrist liaison, but omits the rather disappointing results of efforts to modify the psychiatric attitudes of primary care doctors. It circles around the crucial issue of motivation. Why have UK psychiatrists drifted into general practice settings?

And what is the quality of motivation among their host GPs? A cynic might take the view that motivation on the primary care side is fuelled simply by a desire for a 'garbage disposal' system for difficult patients. There is also the possibility, not denied in the paper, that the price of the model offered might be a lowering of care standards for more chronic and less glamorous patients. It will here be noted that all the data with a bearing on these troublesome issues are, by their nosocomial nature, capable of interpretation in a number of ways. In the end, the pros and cons of the integration argument come down to matters of opinion.

The case for GP–psychiatrist liaison was developed over 20 years ago. This arose from the demonstration of the huge burden of care attributable to minor psychiatric morbidity (and co-morbidity), coupled with the logistic impossibility of catering for this with limited psychiatric resources: administrative and therapeutic logic alike dictated that the challenge be met not by further redeployment of scarce psychiatric resources, but by strengthening the therapeutic effectiveness of GPs themselves. It is a tribute not only to the inherent logic of this argument, but also to the influence of the Maudsley school, that articulate oppostion to this view has not materialised. But other medical specialists could, if they wished, also point to a vast burden of covert and badly managed morbidity in primary care. They have not done so, and there has been no headlong rush of physicians, surgeons, or gynaecologists into GP settings. And why not? Can it be, as has been suggested, that psychiatry has lost its way? Have the two primary responsibilities of mental health services been forgotten in the fascination with legions of potential patients, identified by their high scores on rating scales? The two dimensions of responsibility alluded to are: (a) high-quality emergency response capacity and (b) sustained, high-standard care for the chronically ill. The data so thoroughly reviewed by Goldberg could mean that a UK-type drift towards GP settings predicates a future psychiatry with little to distinguish it from social work. Furthermore, excessive zeal in accepting the integration viewpoint could de-intellectualise psychiatry, just as advances in cognate disciplines have picked up speed to the point where the psychiatrist-scientist is once more in demand.

All this is not to deny that some degree of GP–psychiatrist integration is desirable and will occur: but it will only do so to the extent that the prevailing political and medical ethos will permit. Some will think that the built-in resistance to change is so strong that it would be better to try to accelerate changes already occurring in medical education. Meanwhile, the scenario depicted by Goldberg is as English as afternoon tea: this publication should consider if its wholesale promotion throughout the EC would be as difficult to implement as it would be unlikely to succeed.

10 Process or outcome approach in the evaluation of psychiatric services

PIERLUIGI MOROSINI and FRANCO VELTRO

This paper examines the problems of mental health services evaluation not only from the general point of view of the methods of health service research, but also from that particular orientation which is known as Quality Assurance or Quality Promotion. The more specific features of Quality Assurance are set out in the appendix to this chapter. In the field of Health Services Evaluation, it is customary to distinguish between structure, process, and outcome evaluation (Donabedian, 1980–85; Williamson, 1982). 'Structure' refers to the resources available and their organisation, 'process' to how things are done, and 'outcome' to the end results of health care in terms of mortality, morbidity, and quality of life. This division reflects the predominantly clinical outlook of its originators. For those who are also involved in planning and management of health services, a more complete subdivision may include cost, resources, performance, process, and outcome, with the further subdivisions shown in Table 10.1. In addition to these basic dimensions, it may be useful to consider separately one further aspect relating both to structure and performance – 'accessibility'.

In this more comprehensive framework, the term 'process evaluation' may refer both to the indications and nature of interventions (the traditional use) on the one hand, and to the qualitative aspects of the managerial organisation on the other.

Cost

It is surprising that data about the cost of psychiatric services are not reported more often and are not generally available. In Italy, data about cost are scanty and unreliable; but huge differences are known to exist in per capita costs (in relation to catchment-area population), in the percentage of the total health budget spent on mental health, and in the distribution of costs between hospital and community services. Table 10.2 refers to two mental health services – those of Sardinia and Tuscany (Rudas *et al*, 1989). The latter

TABLE 10.1
Basic components of health services evaluation

Component	Relevant question
(1) Cost	How much is spent?
(2) Structure, sub-divided into:	
2.1 Resources available	What can be used?
2.2 Management	How are things organised?
(3) Process, subdivided into:	
3.1 Performance or amount of interventions	How much is done?
3.2 Quality process, i.e. indications and nature of interventions	How are things done?
(4) Outcome, sub-divided into:	
4.1 Instrumental outcomes	How are the biological/psychological features of clients/users/patients modified in the short term?
4.2 Final outcome	How are the health and quality of life of clients/users/patients modified in the long term?
4.3 Patients'/clients'/users' satisfaction, as a form of both instrumental and final outcome	
(5) Accessibility and acceptability (a component which is not independent, but includes features of both structure and process)	
5.1 service-based items, e.g. opening hours, average waiting time	
5.2 population-based items, e.g. incidence rates, use of private and outside services	

is generally considered among the best community-orientated mental health services in Italy. These few data suffice to give an idea of the general underfinancing of psychiatric services in Italy, and to show how much of the available resources are still devoted to institutional care in some areas. In general, more than 50% of the total budget still goes to the old psychiatric hospitals or to 'contracted out' beds in private psychiatric hospitals.

It is difficult to understand why costs per capita and the distribution of costs among programmes have been so neglected in descriptions of the mental health services of different nations of similar economic status, although it must be acknowledged that comparison of costs is not a simple matter, because of differences in the scope of psychiatric services and in budgeting procedures. This discussion refers to the general costing of psychiatric services, and not to specific studies of cost-effectiveness (see contributions by Knapp and O'Donnell in this volume) which also take into account indirect and non-monetary costs. Häfner & an der Heiden (1989) have provided additional information about the distribution of costs among types of patients and between community and hospital care.

TABLE 10.2
Cost of mental health services for adults in two Italian health districts, 1986

	Health District 10, Sardinia	Health District 23, Tuscany
Total cost per capita population: $	22.0	22.0 (14)[1]
% of total health budget	3.5	2.5 (1.8)[1]
% of mental health budget for private hospitals	43.9	0.0
% for domiciliary care	0.0	10.0
% for old in-patients in public psychiatric hospital	Not included	35.0

1. If the costs for old psychiatric in-patients are excluded, the costs of the Sardinia district were unchanged, while the per capita adult population costs of the Tuscany district decreased to 14 dollars (1.8% of the total health budget).

Resources

It must be emphasised that certain amounts and types of resources are a necessary, if not sufficient condition for the provision of community-orientated psychiatric services of an acceptable standard. Not only the number but also the type and abilities of the staff are of the utmost importance in a comprehensive mental health service, where special skills in social work, occupational therapy, behavioural rehabilitation, and short-term psychotherapy are required. Since the social and behavioural aspects are important in mental health, the layout and decoration of facilities should also be considered: common guidelines should be developed to judge the quality of the physical environment and available equipment, e.g. by developing a check-list and by assessment of videotapes. Not only the resources of the service, but also those of the relevant catchment area should be considered, since the success of rehabilitation efforts depends greatly on the available opportunities for accommodation and jobs. The main elements of psychiatric services resources and some indicators relating to them are listed below:

(a) Items of service delivered (out-patients visits, home visits, day care and day hospital attendances, compulsory admissions, voluntary admissions, miles travelled).
(b) Users and their characteristics (age, sex, 'new' or 'old', diagnoses, social functioning. Are standard definitions of current users followed?).
(c) Type of intervention (psychoactive drugs consumption by category, group and individual psychotherapy sessions performed, group and individual rehabilitation sessions performed, patients transported to day care centres).

Main indicators of the workload of community services
  (a) Current users.
  (b) Staff involved.
  (c) Home visits/involved staff.
  (d) Residents/staff in residential care facilities (staff in full-time equivalents).

Main indicators of hospital performance
  (a) Average length of stay.
  (b) Turnover interval.
  (c) Occupancy rate.
  (d) Hospital admissions/involved staff.

Main indicators concerning users
  (a) Rate of incident and prevalent users by age.
  (b) Sex, diagnosis (percentage distributions are not enough).
  (c) Social functioning levels (in the future).

Management

The coordination of different professions and continuity of care are more important in psychiatry than in most other health fields. It is, for instance, necessary to assess whether and how the hospital and community parts of the service are integrated (separate or rotating staff, a single director, a coordinator of two or more services, etc.). The main elements of the managerial component are listed below:

  (a) Use of other public facilities inside the catchment area (neurology department, 'contracted out' psychiatrists).
  (b) Use of private facilities inside the catchment area (private psychiatric hospitals, private psychiatrists and psychologists).
  (c) Use of public and private facilities outside the catchment area (long-stay patients in psychiatric hospitals outside the catchment area).
  (d) Use of forensic services.
  (e) Destitute people with severe psychiatric disorders.

Indirect indicators
Incidence rates of schizophrenic disorders compared to similar catchment areas.

Performance and accessibility

The main items of performance are listed below:

Of the service
  (a) Type, qualifications, and number of staff (scope of professions, staff turnover, staff age distribution, are "cooperatives" workers included?, is staff expressed in full-time equivalents?).
  (b) Out-patient departments/mental health centres (opening hours, space distribution between common activities rooms and individual consulting rooms, kitchens and canteens in mental health centres, night beds in mental health centres, building and furniture appearance).
  (c) Psychiatric beds in general hospitals (is there a separate psychiatric unit?, beds per room, bathrooms per bed, common activities spaces, access to green spaces, building and furniture appearances).
  (d) Community day care (places in day centres, places in day hospitals, building and furniture appearance).
  (e) 'Cooperatives' for users (numbers employed and kind of work).
  (f) Residential care in the community (number of places for residential care distinguished according to the amount of staff presence and supervision, layout of building, e.g. subdivision in self-contained units for 2–4 people, furniture appearance).
  (g) Transport facilities (cars for staff use, vans for users' transport).
  (h) Beds in private psychiatric hospitals.
  (i) 'Grey' beds, i.e. beds used for psychiatric patients in institutions or departments that are not officially designated for them.

Of the area
  (a) Accommodation opportunities for low-income persons.
  (b) Work opportunities for unskilled persons.

Indicators of resources
  (a) Psychiatric acute beds per 10 000 population.
  (b) Total opening hours of out-patient department per 10 000 population.
  (c) Community psychiatric nurses and social workers per 10 000 population.
  (d) Percentage distribution of different professions.
  (e) Residential care places per 10 000 population.
  (f) Day hospital and day centre places per 10 000 population.
  (g) Ratio of acute psychiatric beds to residential care places.

The main items of accessibility are:

(a) Boundaries, 'coterminality' of various service parts.
(b) Management structure at district and unit level.
(c) Special services for adolescent psychiatry; substance abuse.
(d) Coordination between acute psychiatric beds and community services (rotation of staff between hospital and community).
(e) Fragmentation/coordination of care among professionals.
(f) Individual care plans (are common goals defined and agreed with a multidisciplinary approach and the exact nature of the contribution of each team member identified?).
(g) Continuity of care.
(h) Privacy and personalisation (individual lockers, personal clothing).
(i) Social, recreational, and rehabilitative activities available in day centres, in day hospitals, and for in-patients.
(j) Consultation patterns for prisons, nursing homes, hostels.
(k) Crisis intervention (weekend and night arrangements, out-of-hours availability of the different professions, multidisciplinary crisis intervention teams, arrangements with police, emergency beds in mental health centres).
(l) Resettlement of long-stay hospital in-patients (are adequate facilities developed?).
(m) Cooperation with voluntary and relatives' organisations (are family members attending as volunteers at mental health centres? Are day care centres and/or residential care centres run by voluntary organisations?).
(n) Information system (problem-orientated at clinical records, ease of retrieval of clinical and social records, case registers).
(o) Relationship with general practitioners and other consultants (medical committee forum for joint discussion, responsibility for patients receiving depot injections).

Striking differences appear when the rates of users and proportions of different activities are compared between different services. These differences may be more marked in Italy than elsewhere, because of the regionalisation of health services and the almost complete lack of national standards for psychiatry.

For instance, the rates of patients receiving a domiciliary visit per 10 000 population have a more than tenfold variation – from 45 to 2 – among health districts in Lombardy (Lombardy Region, 1988) (Fig. 10.1). In the UK, the corresponding rates in 5 areas with a psychiatric case register varied from 90 (Nottingham) to 21 (Salford) (Gibbons *et al*, 1984). Psychiatric case registers reveal a considerable variation in incidence and prevalence rates and even more in rates of new long-stay patients. Incidence rates are probably the best indicators of accessibility of services; rates for psychotic problems

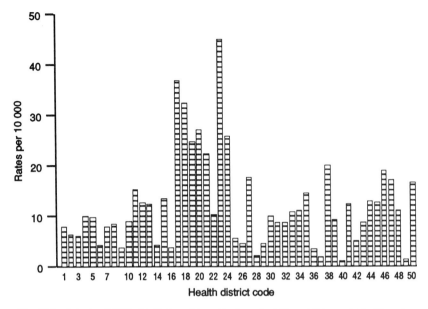

Fig. 10.1. Rates per 10 000 of patients receiving at least one domiciliary visit by mental health services by health districts (coded by number) (Lombardy, 1987)

should be relatively uniform, while those for neurotic disorders reflect more the acceptability of the public service.

The following figures have no claim to be very accurate, but may serve as a frame of reference, to which the correct figures could eventually be related. A European Community Comprehensive Mental Health Service should have an annual prevalence of at least 300 psychotic patients per 100 000 adult population (organic states excluded) of whom at least 30 should be new cases (annual incidence rate); 3 cases per 100 000 population may be expected to be new, severely disturbed patients, who will need some kind of residential care for long periods.

Process evaluation

From both clinical and epidemiological perspectives, the most important components of health service evaluation are, firstly, process and – even more important – outcome. Process evaluation, as now recommended in Quality Assurance programmes, requires the previous consensus on explicit measurable criteria of care, i.e. a previous agreement on how the health professional should behave towards a well-defined health problem. These criteria may concern drugs (indication, dosage, duration), psychological and social interventions, level of care, patterns of follow-up, etc. This requirement explains why process evaluation studies are so difficult in psychotherapy, and almost as problematic in psychiatric rehabilitation. However, the approach known as 'Measurement of needs' offers an interesting solution: it will be discussed below. Many process evaluation studies have been performed on the use of psychotropic drugs, but the criteria may not be easy to agree upon in that field either.

The criteria proposed by Molnar & Feeney (1985) do not include indications for prescriptions, as is common in other Quality Assurance studies (Feldman *et al*, 1983). Another original approach to process evaluation has been developed by the Australian Quality Assurance Project. A questionnaire has been sent to all Australian psychiatrists, asking their treatment recommendations for a number of 'vignettes' which describe cases of depression or schizophrenia (Quality Assurance Project, 1983; 1984).

Outcome evaluation

Outcome evaluation studies concern the assessment of effectiveness, i.e. the routine capacity of health services to improve the health conditions of their users, in contrast to the experimental assessment in randomised controlled trials of efficacy, i.e. the effect of specific health intervention in optimal conditions. Palmer & Nesson (1982) state that outcome evaluation should be preferred to process evaluation when the following conditions apply:

(a) A lack of consensus among professionals about the indications for and types of appropriate intervention.
(b) Complexity of patterns of care and difficulty in clarifying the roles of individual types of intervention.
(c) A focus on evaluation of whole areas, rather than on individual departments or professionals.
(d) A need for a screening tool (see 'sentinel events' below), to be followed by process studies.

Outcome evaluation studies are subject to observational biases, which in mental health may be even more frequent and severe than in other health fields. These may be summarised as follows:

(a) Lack of reliability and accuracy in the definition of diagnoses, degree of severity, and individual prognostic factors, which causes uncertainty about the comparability of groups. However, remarkable progress has been made in this field in recent years.
(b) Greater influence of external factors, e.g. family attitudes and occupational opportunities.

(c) Observer bias, which is more marked for the 'soft' variables often involved in mental health. A particular form of this is 'attention' bias, which can cause an apparent fall in patients' level of social functioning after the beginning of a research project, because staff become more sensitive to previously unnoticed gaps in the subjects' social repertoire.
(d) Complexity of intervention patterns: i.e. difficulty in identifying the specific elements responsible for the differences in outcome.
(e) Discontinuity of the observed effectiveness. This may happen when, at the beginning of a new programme, its enthusiastic advocates achieve excellent results that wane or disappear with the fading of enthusiasm or change of staff.

If the evidence about efficacy remains unconvincing, the best research approach is the randomised controlled trial. However, the cultural and practical difficulties in planning and implementing randomised trials in psychiatry are directly proportional to their interest: relatively easy for new drugs, difficult for different methods of psychotherapy and rehabilitation, and very difficult for community versus hospital care, although some such have been done (Hoult *et al*, 1983). Cochrane's (1972) opinion that clinical trials seem particularly difficult in Catholic countries is no longer true in other fields of medicine, but may still have some relevance when the psychoanalytically orientated training of therapists conflicts with their religious beliefs.

It is useful to distinguish four types of outcome studies. The first is the systematic identification and analysis of sentinel events. The second type is the routine study performed by professionals for their own self-evaluation purposes; these are relatively uncommon, even though interesting methods and tools are now available. However, a valuable approach is the assessment of the attainment of measurable objectives for individual patients (Guy & Moore, 1983). Short rating scales of outcome, such as the ones devised by Green & Gracely (1987) or proposed by Hawk & Carpenter (1975), should become routine in mental health services, and perhaps be incorporated into the data collection of psychiatric registers. Because of improved levels of literacy, self-completed questionnaires on disability and family burden (Weissman, 1981; Morosini *et al*, 1991) as well as patients' self-rating schedules, may also come into general use (Greenfield & Atkinson, 1989).

The third type of outcome study is the mortality study (Tsuang & Simyson, 1985; Bacigalupi *et al*, 1988; Casadebaig *et al*, 1990). Mortality rates are a very crude indicator of outcome, but are relatively easy to collect. Large-scale historical studies on cohorts of patients recruited many years ago may make useful contributions towards the evaluation of community care in different countries. The fourth type of outcome study comprises more ambitious studies, with careful selection of subjects, reliable methodology, and independence of observers, such as the ones at Friern Hospital, London (see Leff, this volume), and in Sydney, Australia (Andrews *et al*, in press) as well as well known studies on the outcome of schizophrenia (Ciompi & Muller, 1980; McGlashan & Carpenter, 1988; Shepherd *et al*, 1989).

Sentinel events

Sentinel events are those outcomes whose occurrence should give rise to *ad hoc* enquiries, aimed at ascertaining what has really happened and whether avoidable factors were involved (Rutstein, 1976). A tentative list of possible sentinel events for mental health services is:

Negative events
   (a) More than two acute crises a year in a young patient.
   (b) Patient who has not left house/room for more than a certain amount of time.
   (c) Loss to follow-up of a patient with a threatening condition.
   (d) Patient jailed.
   (e) Suicide after discharge within a defined period.
   (f) Hostile family attitudes.
   (g) Development of alcohol dependence.
   (h) Fall with injury.
   (i) Assault against other patients or staff.
   (j) Discharge against medical advice.

Positive events
   (a) Return to satisfactory full employment of an unemployed schizo-phrenic patient.
   (b) Independent satisfactory living achieved by a former long-term psychiatric in-patient.

They could be recorded by psychiatric case registers, which have been criticised for not giving information on quality of care. In the mental health field, 'sentinel' items may be defined not only for outcome but also for structure (e.g. lack of vocational training) and for process (e.g. refusal to visit a possible patient at home, or lack of support or educational programmes for schizophrenic patients' relatives). The development of positive sentinel events might also be envisaged, e.g. the return to full, unsheltered employment for an unemployed schizophrenic patient.

Satisfaction

Patients' and relatives' satisfaction are kinds of outcome that are receiving ever-increasing attention in the mental health field. They are more concerned with the availability and accessibility of services and patient–professional interaction than the technical competence of health professionals. Routinely self-completed questionnaires may also be successful for this aspect of evaluation.

Measurement of needs

An exceptionally interesting approach which combines elements of process and outcome evaluation for the long-term mentally ill has recently been proposed by the MRC Social Psychiatry Research Unit in London (Brewin & Wing, 1988; Brewin *et al*, 1988). Needs are defined on the basis of problems in individual areas of functioning, rather than diagnostic labels: a need is present where a patient's functioning falls below or threatens to fall below some minimum specified level and this is due to some remediable or potentially remediable cause. The authors seem to have succeeded in obtaining a significant consensus from rehabilitation and medical staff about what constitutes an adequate intervention for meeting the unmet needs. The wishes and attitudes of the patients are taken into account. Outcome evaluation is present in the evaluation of unmet needs, while process evaluation almost unavoidably follows when the remedial actions, to be implemented according to a predefined set of criteria, are decided upon.

Future international evaluative studies

The aim of international evaluative studies should no longer be simple description, but the promotion of change towards the best possible practice. There is a wide spectrum of possible approaches that have different organisational difficulties, research contents, and time spans, but all seem potentially effective.

Resources, organisation, and performance evaluation

Exchanges of advisory visits, as performed by the UK Health Advisory Service (NHS, 1989) and the Dutch Hospital Board (Hardeman, 1988), may represent the best approach for this component. It is necessary, however, to develop explicit guidelines on the procedures to be followed during the visits and also, if possible, to agree a list of minimum standards. This could profit from US, Canadian, and Australian experiences on accreditation of mental health services (Canadian Council on Hospital Accreditation, 1986; Australian Council on Health Care Standards, 1990).

The development of such guidelines and minimum standards and the study of the feasibility of their application might in itself represent a useful quality assurance exercise; the research interest lies in assessment of the amount of agreement obtainable and in evaluation of the impact of the advisory visits. Items of process evaluation can be included in advisory visits, e.g. auditing of quality of the clinical records and of the use of psychotropic drugs.

Process evaluation

In this field, an international study of the prescription and use of psychotropic drugs might prove of great practical benefit.

Outcome evaluation

Two main options are possible:

(a) Development of common, easy-to-administer tools for self-evaluation of patients and their relatives, and the application of these to large cohorts in a number of centres. This approach is less scientifically valid than the following one, but perhaps more effective in promoting change.
(b) Cohort studies of carefully selected groups of new cases, with consideration of all known prognostic factors. Precise criteria for the choice of services to be compared should also be developed.

'Need' assessment

This approach seems very promising for comparison of the services for long-term severely mentally ill patients. There are undoubtedly a number of obstacles in the way of its application in an international setting (for instance, avoiding selection biases may prove difficult); however, it seems the best way at present to promote both a common way of thinking and an acceptable level of practice everywhere.

Appendix: Quality assurance in mental health

A comprehensive survey of the Quality Assurance (QA) approach in psychiatry has been made by Fauman (1989), although its main focus is on the US scene. The main concepts of Health Services Quality Assurance are briefly summarised here. Some of the definitions used are original, but consistent with their practical use in QA and, it is hoped, more operational and unambiguous.

Problem, criteria, indicator, threshold, sentinel events

A problem may be defined as an opportunity to improve care. Explicit criteria are measurable statements that define appropriate clinical care; they may apply to the structure, performance, process, or outcome of care, and serve as a yardstick against which the actual care can be evaluated. Explicit criteria should be stated in operational terms, and be based on a critical review of the relevant scientific literature or on expert opinion – but only when the scientific evidence is inadequate. They should be accepted by the professionals involved in the QA activities. In some cases, explicit criteria may be used to screen out cases to be reviewed 'implicitly' by panels of experts. For instance, a criterion for the pharmacological treatment of depression may state that patients with a major depressive disorder should be given 100–200 mg daily of a tricyclic antidepressant, such as imipramine, for at least two weeks.

Indicators may be considered as criteria that can be collected routinely, and so monitored in a continuous way. The difference between criteria and indicators depends on the available information system. Negative indicators may also be called 'sentinel events', according to Rutstein (1976).

A *threshold*, or 'standard' in QA terminology, is the percentage of times that the relevant criterion or indicator has to be fulfilled in order for one to be satisfied with the quality of care, or, if the criterion or indicator is negative, to suspect or conclude that the quality of care can be improved. Some negative indicators, such as suicide in a recently discharged patient, may have a threshold of 0%, so that all instances of such suicides are to be reviewed. However, in most cases, to put a threshold at 0 or 100% is unrealistic, because this does not take into account both the unavoidable rigidity of the criterion, compared to the complexity and variability of clinical disorders, and the poor cost-effectiveness of improving an already high level of care.

Thresholds may be normative, i.e. defined by expert opinion, or empirical, i.e. based on statistical distributions. An empirical (statistically derived) threshold for a performance indicator may be that only 5% of admissions to a certain psychiatric department in a general hospital should have a length of stay longer than 21 days – 21 days being the 95% percentile of the statistical distribution of lengths of stay in all psychiatric departments in that particular region. A normative (professionally derived) threshold may be that the proportion of patients discharged against medical advice should not exceed 4% (1 out of 25), because this level is thought to be still tolerable and not needing *ad hoc* investigation.

It has been repeatedly emphasised that the ultimate target of quality assurance monitoring is the resolution of identified problems, and that the collection of data is not an end in itself. A QA project includes the following steps:

(a) Identification of problems (e.g. through the monitoring of a set of indicators).
(b) Selection of the problem to be checked first (the one where improvements may result in the greatest benefits for the users).
(c) Explicit definition of criteria, if they are not yet available, or discussion as to whether they need updating.
(d) Planning and implementation of a study to assess the amount and cause of any discrepancies between care received and the criteria involved.
(e) Modifying intervention (organisational change, in-service training, etc).
(f) Assessment of the impact of the intervention.

The QA cycle may then begin again, from steps (c) to (f), if the problem under examination has not been satisfactorily solved, or from steps (a) or (b) with a new problem.

Identification

The psychiatric conditions deserving of priority for QA activities should be the following:

(a) The most frequent.
(b) The most severe and disabling.
(c) The most amenable to effective intervention.

It would be interesting, however, to study the degree of agreement among psychiatrists in selecting disorders according to these criteria.

Process and outcome

The US Joint Commission for Accreditation of Health Care Organizations (JCHCO) has stated that it expects to concentrate more on outcomes measurement in the future (JCHCO, 1989); process evaluation should be limited to those elements of care that have clearly been shown to be directly related to clinical outcome. The new approach emphasised the development of indicators to monitor high-volume or high-risk areas of practice. The JCHCO will ask whether the organisation being evaluated provides high-quality care, rather than whether it has the capacity to provide it (Faumann, 1989). This approach is consistent with the main trend in quality assurance during the past 20 years, which is away from time-consuming, mainly retrospective medical record audits to flexible monitoring of important variables related to the outcome of care. The JCHCO has developed pilot indicators for general hospital care (JCHCO, 1989), but not yet for mental health services.

References

ANDREWS, G., TEESSON, M., STEWART, G. W., *et al* (1991) Community placement of the chronic mentally ill. *Hospital and Community Psychiatry* (in press).
AUSTRALIAN COUNCIL ON HEALTH CARE STANDARDS (1990) *The Accreditation Guide* (8th edn). Sydney: ACHCS.
BACIGALUPI, M., CECERE, F., ARCA', M., *et al* (1988) La mortalità dei recoverati negli ospedali psichiatrici pubblici della Regione Lazio: primi risultati. *Epidemiologia e Prevenzione*, **35**, 11–16.
BREWIN, C. R. & WING, J. K. (1988) Manual of the MRC Needs for Care Assessments. Unpublished Manuscript. Institute of Psychiatry, London.
——, ——, MANGEN, S., *et al* (1988) Needs for care among the long-term mentally ill: a report from the Camberwell High Contact Survey. *Psychological Medicine*, **18**, 457–468.
CANADIAN COUNCIL ON HOSPITAL ACCREDITATION (1986) *Guide to Accreditation of Canadian Mental Health Centres*. Ottawa: CCHA.
CASADEBAIG, F., QUEMSADA, N. & CHEVALIER, A. (1990) Évolution de la mortalité des malades mentaux. *Revue Epidemiologie et Santé Publique*, **39**, 227–236.
CIOMPI, L. & MULLER, C. (1980) Catamnestic long-term study on the course of life and ageing of schizophrenics. *Schizophrenia Bulletin*, **6**, 606–618.
COCHRANE, A. L. (1972) *Effectiveness and Efficiency: Random Reflections on Health Services*. London: Nuffield Provincial Hospital Trust.
DONABEDIAN, A. (1980–85) *Explorations in Quality assessment and Monitoring*. Vol. I, 1980; vol. II, 1982; vol. III, 1985. Ann Arbor, MI: Health Administration Press.
FAUMAN, M. A. (1989) Quality assurance monitoring in psychiatry. *American Journal of Psychiatry*, **146**, 1121–1130.

FELDMAN, J., WILNER, S. & WINICKOFF, R. (1983) A study of lithium carbonate use in a health maintenance organization. *Quality Review Bulletin*. Special Edition: *Quality Assurance in Mental Health*, pp. 33–38.

GIBBONS, J. L., JENNINGS, C. & WING, J. K. (1984) *Psychiatric Care in Eight Register Areas. Statistics from Eight Psychiatric Case Registers in Great Britain*. Southampton Psychiatric Case Register, Knowle Hospital.

GREEN, R. & GRACELY, E. (1987) A review of outcome assessment tools. *Community Mental Health Journal*, **23**, 81–102.

GREENFIELD, I. K. & ATKINSON, C. C. (1989) Steps toward a multifactorial satisfaction scale for primary care and mental health services. *Evaluation and Program Planning*, **5**, 278–286.

GUY, M. & MOORE, L. S. (1983) The Goal Attainment Scale for psychiatric in-patients. *Quality Review Bulletin*. Special Edition: *Quality Assurance in Mental Health*, pp. 17–27.

HARDEMAN, W. J. (1988) *Quality and Efficiency in Mental Hospitals: Discussion Paper*. Utrecht: National Hospital Board.

HAWK, A. B. & CARPENTER, W. T. (1975) Diagnostic criteria and five-year outcome in schizophrenia. *Archives of General Psychiatry*, **32**, 343–347.

HÄFNER, H. & VAN DER HEIDEN, W. (1989) The evaluation of mental health care systems. *British Journal of Psychiatry*, **155**, 12–17.

HOULT, J., REYNOLDS, I., CHARBONNEAU-PARIS, M., *et al* (1983) Psychiatric hospital versus community treatment: the results of a randomized trial. *Australian and New Zealand Journal of Psychiatry*, **17**, 160–167.

JOINT COMMISSION FOR ACCREDITATION OF HEALTH CARE ORGANIZATIONS (1989) *Consolidated Standard Manual*. Chicago: Joint Commission for Accreditation of Health Care Organizations.

LOMBARDY REGION (1988) *Coordinamento per i Servizi Sociali. Progetto-obiettivo. Tutela sociosanitaria dei malati di mente: sistema informativo*. Milano: Settore al Coordinamento per i Servizi Sociali Regione Lombardia.

McGLASHAN, T. H. & CARPENTER, W. T. (eds) (1988) Long-term follow-up studies of schizophrenia. *Schizophrenia Bulletin*, **14**, 497–707.

MOLNAR, G. & FEENEY, M. G. (1985) Computer-assisted review of antipsychotics in acute care units. *Quality Review Bulletin*, September, 271–274.

MOROSINI, P. L., VELTRO, F., RONCONE, R., *et al* (1991) *Di un questionario per la Valutazione del Carico e dell'atteggiamento dei Familiari*. L'Aquila: Proceedings of the II Congress of the Italian Society for Psychosocial Rehabilitation.

NATIONAL HEALTH SERVICE HEALTH ADVISORY SERVICE (1989) *Annual Report 1987–1988*. Sutton, (Survey): NHSNAS.

PALMER, R. H. & NESSON, H. R. (1982) A review of methods for ambulatory medical care evaluations. *Medical Care*, **20**, 758–778.

QUALITY ASSURANCE PROJECT (1983) Treatment outlines for the management of schizophrenics. *Australian and New Zealand Journal of Psychiatry*, **17**, 129–146.

—— (1984) Treatment outlines for the management of schizophrenics. *Australian and New Zealand Journal of Psychiatry*, **18**, 19–38.

RUDAS, N., CARPINIELLO, B., CARTA, M., *et al* (1989) *Dieci anni di assistenza psichiatrica territoriale. Progressi in Psichiatria. Standard diagnostici ed epidemiologici*. Roma: CIC Edizioni Internationali. 200–223.

RUTSTEIN, D. (1976) Measuring the quality of medical care: a clinical method. *New England Journal of Medicine*, **294**, 582–588.

SHEPHERD, M., WATT, D., FALLOON, I., *et al* (1989) The natural history of schizophrenia: a five-year follow-up study. *Psychological Medicine* (monograph suppl. 15).

TSUANG, M. A. & SIMYSON, J. (1985) Mortality studies in psychiatry. Should they stop or proceed? *Archives of General Psychiatry*, **42**, 98–103.

WEISSMAN, M. M., SHOLOMSKAS, D. & JOHN, K. (1981) The assessment of social adjustment by patient self-report. *Archives of General Psychiatry*, **33**, 1111–1115.

WILLIAMSON, J. W. (1982) *Teaching Quality Assurance and Cost Containment in Health Care*. San Francisco, CA: Jossey Boss.

11 The direct costs of the community care of chronically mentally ill people

MARTIN KNAPP

To the practitioner working in the mental health field, it may seem as if the words 'cost' and 'care' feature in the same sentence with increasing and alarming frequency. The two do not look like comfortable bedfellows. Policies directed at the management of costs must seem to many people directly to threaten service practices dominated by considerations of the quality or consequences of care. Yet, it must also seem as if every new clinical or practice suggestion today must run the gauntlet of a series of cost questions which are, at best, inconvenient, and sometimes simply terminal.

In many European and other countries, the appearance of the cost dimension (on more than an occasional basis) in public policy debates and pronouncements followed hard on the heels of the worldwide economic depression of the 1970s which stemmed from the rapid oil price inflation. In the years that have followed, different sets of political, ideological, professional, and other forces in each of these countries have shaped slightly different policy responses to these economic problems. There are, of course, similarities, one of them being the link between fiscal constraint and policies of deinstitutionalisation. Although the modern-day preference for the community location of long-term heath and social care for this client group stems from arguments and evidence couched in terms of clinical and social outcomes, and/or in terms of basic human rights, community care has been enthusiastically embraced by the 'fiscal hawks' in government. It is rare, of course, for these 'hawks' to find themselves in the position of advocating on financial grounds precisely the kind of policy which finds favour for quite different reasons with a majority of key health and social care professionals. In some of the member countries of the EC, the fiscal encouragement of community care may not have been of great importance, or even evident at all, but it appears to have happened often enough to prompt us to ask whether the encouragement is really for the best.

This is not the only relevant international similarity. In the present context, it is possible to draw international parallels in the developing attitudes and behaviour of those service professionals and managers who must act on political directives which have been greatly influenced by the hawks and their predatory tendencies. Their reactions move through a common series of phases, which help to explain at least three things: (a) why there is comparatively little evidence on the costs of mental health services; (b) why much of that evidence is unreliable, either in construction or utilisation; and (c) why we now have an excellent opportunity to do better.

Within the public services generally – and the mental health care sector has been no exception – the inevitable initial reaction to the downward trend in public spending is most commonly one of hostility. This takes many forms, including the outright refusal to implement any practices or take any initiatives which will cut spending, energetic lobbying for a return to the halcyon days of another era when resources grew faster than needs (in the UK this was the early 1970s), and the denigration of any attempt to place such initiatives on a sounder evidential base.

This first reaction – the 'rubbishing' phase – is commonly followed by panic. As opposition to austere macroeconomic policies began to wane – partly out of exhaustion in the face of continuing spending constraints, partly from the realisation that these constraints were not transitory, and partly because of a general drift to the political right, it was replaced by a kind of frenetic and seemingly irrational behaviour. In this case, however, the behaviour was corporate. Faced with the directive to deliver equivalent (or better) services at lower (or equivalent) cost, service managers or policy-makers were to be observed unselectively grabbing every snippet of cost evidence. If the 'rubbishing' of attempts to infuse mental health care policy with cost arguments has not succeeded in changing the general direction of policy, and if the hasty and uncritical conflation of previously available data succeeds only in generating more heat than light, the third phase should be the sponsorship of new evidence and the construction of new argument. Again, concentrating on the cost dimension is characterised by, *inter alia*, a much higher profile for the economist.

Economics has as its principal focus the study of scarcity – it is no surprise that the discipline has been labelled ''the dismal science'' – and has thus both accumulated experience and developed comparative advantage in the design and execution of cost research. Economists are as fallible as anyone else, but there is also the problem that their involvement is commonly too little, too late or too remote. For instance, a policy-maker or clinical researcher may recognise that cost insights are helpful and that extant data are insufficient, but may be able only to 'tack' new costs evidence on to, e.g. evidence on the clinical outcomes of alternative service options, as an afterthought. Or it may only be possible – because of funding constraints, research management considerations, or the politics of scientific publishing – for the economic study to be conducted and reported at arm's length from the study of clinical outcomes. Or it may be that there are no economists sufficiently skilled, accessible, or congenial to include in the research team.

The procedure which is much to be preferred is the premeditated and purposive integration of costs with the other research dimensions. This means not only the regular interchange of ideas, data, results, and interpretations, but also the construction and testing of hypotheses which are not 'cost questions' or 'clinical outcome questions', but the types of question faced by the policy-maker who has to balance resources against achievements or efficiency against equity. Many of today's policy questions, raised in the 'construction phase', cannot be answered by economists, or psychiatrists, or medical sociologists, or psychologists, or statisticians, but only by combinations of people with these skills.

Four rules for costs research

There are four simple rules to observe in the costing of mental health services. Firstly, costs should be comprehensively measured, in that they range over all relevant service and other components of the care 'packages' under consideration. Secondly, the cost variations that are inevitably revealed in any empirical exercise – variations among patients, facilities, areas of the country, etc. – should not be glossed over or relegated to a table of standard deviations. The variations offer a wealth of information which, if handled properly, provides numerous policy and practice insights. These variations immediately encourage comparisons – this service is 'cheaper' than that one, this group of patients is 'more costly' to accommodate than that group, this hospital is 'less efficient' than another – and we must urge caution when making these comparisons. This cautionary note is the third of the costing rules: specifically, only like-with-like comparisons have full validity, even though insights can be retrieved from less-than-perfect comparisons. Finally, in the discussion and analysis of policy, cost information should not stand in isolation from other relevant evidence: costs should be integrated with information on patient outcomes for the purposes of most kinds of evaluative investigation. Sole reliance on cost findings is going to be scientifically acceptable only under special circumstances, even if it has political acceptability. Equally, of course, neglecting costs when making policy decisions, or when undertaking the evaluations which inform them, should also prompt questions about scientific validity.

These four rules are, in fact, no different in intent from the basic principles of any evaluation; they tell us to measure comprehensively the effects, exploit and explore intersubject variations, carefully define control or comparison groups, and avoid viewing the findings in isolation from other relevant factors or perspectives. Costs research, in its intentions and execution, requires no dramatic departure from previous principles. The four rules for a good costing study provide the framework for this paper, and in subsequent sections recent economic enquiries are employed to illustrate how these rules may be followed in practice and what consequences may follow from ignoring or breaking them.

I am unable to offer a fully comprehensive review of every piece of cost research on long-term mental health services that has been undertaken in the EC. I am familiar with the state of research on the economics of mental health care in only a few countries or areas within the EC, while for those countries with which I *am* familiar, it would be hard, for reasons associated almost exclusively with the previously posited phasing of interest in costs, to engage in positive and constructive debate. Two of the purposes of a workshop such as this must be to broaden the international baseline for research activities and generalisations and to challenge academic or geographical isolation.

The comprehensive costs of long-term care

Why go comprehensive?

Of those people with a chronic mental illness who are in contact with a health or social services agency, the majority would be receiving more than one care or support service, probably from more than one agency. A resident of a local authority hostel may be regularly visited by a community psychiatric nurse (CPN), may attend a voluntary organisation's day centre, may occasionally see a psychiatrist at a hospital out-patient clinic, and may enjoy some income support from the social security branch of government. Any evaluation of local authority hostels, CPNs, voluntary-sector day care, hospital psychiatry, or income support programmes which seeks to consider the resource dimension should, in principle, include every one of these service inputs. Even if the aim of an evaluation is simply to compare the costs of local authority and private sector hostel accommodation, it would be dangerous to define costs so narrowly as to exclude these other services. The reason for this is that the combinations of services received by any one person tend not to be thrown together willy-nilly. In this instance it is likely that the staff of a local authority hostel 'network' in different ways from the staff of a private hostel; for instance, they may have better links with the health service but less access to day-care provision. Correlation between services is one of the underlying principles of case management, and the onward march of this approach to individual care planning is one of the most irresistible phenomena in the socio-medical services of many countries.

There is another reason for adhering to the comprehensiveness rule. Consider the comparison of long-term hospital residence and community care. To make a sensible comparison, the costs of the latter would need to be defined so as to range widely over all manner of services, because hospital budgets – which would be the starting point for the costing of the former – are so inclusive, covering most facets of accommodation, day-to-day living costs, treatment, social activities, and employment. The rationale for comprehensiveness in this case is now that it is easier to work with current budgeting conventions for the hospital sector, and to measure community costs so as to achieve consistency of coverage than it is to attempt to disaggregate hospital accounts so as to conform with some definition of 'community'. Not only would such a definition be arbitrary in most cases, but the disaggregation of gross hospital costs, e.g. into accommodation and treatment components would be extremely difficult to effect. The alternative task of comprehensively costing every element of community care is not easy either (cf. Dickey *et al*, 1986), but it is probably the lesser of the two evils.

The comprehensive costing of mental health services raises a number of conceptual and practical issues; it is also controversial. For example, it has been pointed out that it is unfair to include daily living expenses, housing rents, and routine visits to the family practitioner in the costs of community care, since every one of us has these basic needs. But only if utilisation of these services is identical for the options being studied is it legitimate to ignore the associated costs.

How comprehensive?

However, there has to be a practical limit to any empirical exercise. For example, chronic mental illness by its very definition implies long-term intervention by health or social care agencies, and yet an evaluation cannot go on for as long as clients receive care before reaching some conclusion about costs (or effects). In some health and social care contexts, there is only a short interval between the start and end dates. By contrast, an evaluation of a care programme for people with chronic mental illness which sought temporal comprehensiveness would have to run from the onset of illness or the beginning of a formal intervention by a care agency until each client in the care programme died, for many of the service decisions taken today are deliberately intended to have life span effects (and others do so in practice). In fact, cost and outcome implications of many policy decisions outlive the clients immediately affected by them, as with the permanent closure of a hospital or the heavy capital investment in new community accommodation. The practical question is, then, to decide over what length of time costs are to be measured, particularly when the services or systems under examination are in transition. Often, the time span decision is taken out of the researcher's hands – a policy decision is imminent – and there is the additional constraint imposed by the convention of annual financial reporting. Nevertheless, in principle, the time dimension to a study is a research parameter.

Perpendicular to the time dimension is the question of which services, activities, and expenditures to include. Should we include the forgone earnings (and associated losses in national productivity) of people with a mental illness, or the burden of informal care falling to relatives or neighbours? Is a social security benefit a cost? There is no simple answer to each of these questions, mainly because of different policy questions and contexts.

A popular academic exercise two or three decades ago was the costing of the broadest economic costs of mental illness *per se*, and especially the effects on gross national product (Fein, 1958; Conley *et al*, 1973). However, the problem under study is so huge that the assumptions under which a costing is undertaken – in particular, the *ceteris paribus* condition – are unlikely to hold, nor is it quite clear what one does with the results. Fewer such problems arise in the costing of foregone earnings or productivity in smaller-scale evaluations, for it is now reasonable to assume that the rest of the economy or society remains largely unaffected as a consequence of policy changes implicit in the evaluation, and there are obvious practical implications. Thus, the productivity benefits (negative or saved costs) flowing from the Training in Community Living programme developed in Madison and replicated elsewhere are an important and manageable component of the evaluation of this service for people with acute mental illness (Weisbrod *et al*, 1980; Weisbrod, 1983). The usual proxy measure for productivity is earnings, which are an indicator of interest in their own right for the purposes of examining the distributional consequences of policy changes. In the UK, Ginsberg & Marks (1977) and Jones *et al* (1980) have taken this route, and the economic evaluation of the Maudsley's Daily Living Programme will do likewise. (The Programme and its general evaluation are described by Marks *et al*, 1988.)

Three caveats should be entered, however, firstly, using earnings as a measure of productivity is valid only under certain theoretically derived conditions, and without detailing these, it is important to note that they may not apply. Secondly, there is the danger that including productivity or earnings in an evaluation "will tend to discriminate against the more seriously ill patients, the young, the retired, minorities and people living in areas of high unemployment" (Hurst, 1988). The discrimination would only follow if economic efficiency (e.g. maximising the return to public expenditure) was the sole objective of government, yet we know that equity or fairness also figures in policy decisions. However, lost productivity costs might easily swamp service costs for some groups of people, and simplistic research conclusions or policy recommendations could then prove discriminatory. Thirdly, in the particular case of patients with chronic psychiatric illness, most are unemployed, or employed only in very low paid 'sheltered' settings, whether or not they are living 'in the community'. If the research brief is to estimate the global costs of such chronic illness – including life chances missed through illness, inappropriate institutionalisation, etc. – these productivity/earnings costs would be included, but most

F

evaluations focus on the comparative merits of alternative service options (e.g. hospital against community care) for which these particular costs could often sensibly be treated only as identical. If there is reason to believe that they are not identical, it is usual to find such dimensions included among the outcomes within an evaluation.

Missed life chances are costs which are not easily reduced to monetary magnitudes. The same is true of the burden borne by informal carers in the community, ranging from day-to-day direct financial support and loss of earnings, to losses of leisure time and general psychological strain. Again, this is a facet of evaluation which is more commonly and conveniently included among the outcomes than the costs – but which is most commonly ignored altogether – and is outside the scope of this paper.

Books on the theory of cost-benefit analysis devote much space to 'transfer payments', i.e., transfers of money not made in return for goods or services. Social security payments come into this category – they move purchasing power from taxpayers to benefit recipients, and the 'cost' to one group is exactly offset, minus the administrative burden, by the gain to the other. In strict aggregate efficiency terms, it would make no difference if benefit levels were doubled or halved, but there are good reasons for retaining an interest in social security payments. Firstly, rather than confining itself to such global aggregates of efficiency, any policy enquiry worth its salt would look at the distributional consequences of alternative courses of action, because the group which is doing the subsidising has generally been larger, more powerful, and less enthusiastic about egalitarianism than the group being subsidised. Secondly, the flow of funds between the health, social care, housing, and income maintenance components of the 'system' supporting people with chronic psychiatric illness create incentives for particular courses of action (in the UK at the present time, such incentives are often of a most perverse kind). There are, then, efficiency implications of redistributive policies, and these are most certainly not route-neutral. Thirdly, in the absence of specific household expenditure data, social security payments have often been used as proxies for the 'living' expenditures of recipients. Since benefit levels in no country with which I am familiar are sufficient to permit the accrual of savings (beyond the short term), these proxies are probably reasonably accurate. (Their accuracy in the UK is validated by comparison with household spending, as recorded in the annual Family Expenditure Survey.) It certainly makes no sense to throw benefit information away, if there are no estimates of daily living expenditure to put in its place.

How are the costs measured?

The cost figure quoted by or obtained from care agencies is either total cost (aggregate spending on a service, usually during one financial year) or average cost (this aggregate divided by some measure of workload, such as the number of clients seen or the number of in-patient bed-days). These are all accounting costs, based as they are on the reported expenditures of agencies. By contrast, economists advocate using marginal opportunity cost, i.e. the addition to total cost attributable to the inclusion of one more client (the production of one more unit of 'output' in general economic contexts), based not on the accounts of money spent, but on opportunities foregone. Marginal opportunity cost is the concept which figures in theoretical discourses about efficiency, but may not be appropriate to problems in the real world.

There is no doubt that marginal cost is intrinsically the correct magnitude to use, but, in practice, reliance is usually placed on average cost. In fact, today's (short run) average revenue cost, plus appropriate capital and overhead elements, is close to the likely long-run marginal cost (LRMC) for most services in this research area. The immediate cost of 'slotting' one more person into day care or accommodating one more resident in a hostel – the short-run marginal cost (SRMC) – is very small. But if national policy intentions are to substitute community services for all or most long-term hospital beds – which is the case in many countries, including at least Spain, Italy, most parts of the UK (Scotland is the exception), Sweden, the USA, and Canada – and if these intentions are to be evaluated, it makes no sense to use the SRMC, since there is an obvious limit to the number of people who can be 'slotted' into extant services. Among the many studies which have taken this route are those by Jones *et al* (1980), Mangen *et al* (1983), and Knapp *et al* (1991). Interestingly, a recent examination of psychiatric hospital in-patient costs found the (short-run) marginal cost to be little different from average revenue cost (see discussion below on 'like-with-like comparisons'), but this proximity is more the exception than the rule.

Opportunity costing endeavours to measure the true private or social value of a resource in its best alternative use, and in a perfectly informed and frictionless market economy, this would be identical to the price paid for the resource in the market-place. But not everything is marketed, not every market works smoothly, and information is rarely complete, with the result that observed prices and opportunity costs diverge. Thus, the recorded depreciation payments on capital equipment or buildings do not usually reflect the opportunity costs of using these durable resources, nor do the (zero) payments to volunteers necessarily indicate their social value. The comprehensive measurement of cost should include the estimation of opportunity cost, and this fundamental principle should never be abandoned, but enthusiasm for the principle generally has to be tempered when it comes to application.

An example of comprehensive costing

In 1983, the UK Department of Health & Social Security announced a demonstration programme to promote and evaluate the development of community care services for people who had been accommodated in hospital for some years, but who probably no longer needed to be there. It was considered that community living could be better for them, but there were few community facilities to receive them. This 'Care in the Community' programme covered a number of long-term care groups (people with chronic mental illness, learning difficulty or mental handicap, physical handicap, or age-related mental ill-health or physical frailty). All of the hospitals from which people moved were run by the National Health Service, while the community services were delivered and coordinated by a variety of public, voluntary, and private agencies. The programme has been evaluated by the PSSRU: the dimensions of the evaluation were many, and included costs and 'welfare' outcomes for those hospital residents who moved to the community (see discussion below on 'merging costs and outcomes').

This study is the largest such examination in the UK to date: it covered 54 hospitals and 28 demonstration projects – based in as many different district health authorities and local authorities – as well as collecting data from and about over 1300 hospital residents, 800 of whom moved to the community, and from and about over 1000 hospital and community staff. Twelve of the projects focused on people with mental health problems, four of which set out to establish community care for elderly people with mental impairments. The other eight projects, from which illustrations will be taken in this paper, were in London (Brent, Greenwich, and Waltham Forest), Buckinghamshire, Chichester, Warrington, West Berkshire and West Lancashire.

Costs were measured comprehensively for both hospital and community settings. Hospital costs were based on average revenue expenditures for whole establishments, though disaggregated for some purposes down to the ward level, plus a capital element (based on a valuation of site and durable resources, as an annuity over 60 years at 5%), plus a small proportion to reflect service inputs from outside the hospital budget, such as social work, education, or volunteer visiting (this proportion was based on research in a small number of the hospitals included in the study). The community costs were based on interviews with staff (often case managers) and were designed to cover every service and item of expenditure for each person over a nine-month period. We developed an instrument specifically for the study – the Client Service Receipt Interview (CSRI) – which has subsequently been used (usually in slightly modified form) in several other studies of mental health services. Social security payments were used as proxies for living expenses, and were also the subject of study in their own right, though not reported here. (See the interim findings in Thomason & Beecham, 1988, and the

TABLE 11.1

Community care cost components for clients in the 'Care in the Community' demonstration programme (Mental Health Projects) as a percentage of total package cost

	% of total cost
Accommodation and living costs	61.0
Project overheads (management) costs	6.3
General practitioner costs	0.4
Other family practitioner committee costs	0.2
Day activity costs	17.3
Education costs	0.9
In-patient hospital residence costs	3.2
Day- and out-patient hospital service costs	1.3
Community nursing costs	1.4
Community medical care costs	1.8
Community social care costs	6.2
Police costs	0
Total percentage	100.0
Average cost per client week (1986–87 prices): £ sterling	271

final conclusions in Knapp *et al*, 1991, Ch. 14.) Conventional opportunity costing principles were adopted as far as possible, and observed average costs were adjusted so as to approach long-run marginal cost values.

The comprehensive costs, expressed in pounds sterling at 1986–87 prices and arranged by the type of accommodation occupied at the time of the collection of the community service utilisation data (approximately nine months after each client left hospital), are summarised in Table 11.1. The largest single component of cost is accommodation, which often includes much of the staff support needed by clients, but 'community care' does not stop there, as the many other service components indicate. It should be noted that (a) comprehensive costing is necessary in order to get a picture of the implications of community care for public, voluntary, and private agencies and for the personal resources of clients; (b) it is also necessary to ensure definitional consistency when making comparisons with hospital, since most of these services have already been subsumed within hospital budgets; and (c) it is feasible to do so.

The first costing rule requires that costs be taken into account whether or not they fall to the agency primarily responsible for delivering or coordinating care. "Unless costs are defined and measured comprehensively, one treatment mode may appear to be less costly than another when in reality that mode merely shifts costs into forms that have not been measured" (Weisbrod *et al*, 1980).

Exploring and exploiting variations

The second rule for a costing study is not to gloss over the (generally quite marked) variations in cost that are uncovered in an empirical study. Implicit in the earlier account of costing principles, and necessary in order to manage the complex task of measuring comprehensive costs is a preference for gathering service utilisation information and for calculating associated costs at the level of the individual service user. This is also the most popular level of disaggregation in clinical evaluations. In both the clinical and economic contexts, it is the intrinsic variation in individual circumstances and needs which generates this preference. Such variation is obviously not random. For this reason, it is only with reservation and in order to summarise a mass of data that the clinical evaluator would refer to the 'average patient'. Certainly, good clinical practice would not ordinarily be based on routinised diagnoses, informed by broad statistical summaries of a central tendency. Generalisations from previous research and hands-on experience would be interpreted and adapted in the light of the specific circumstances of each individual case. For exactly analogous reasons, we should regard with suspicion those policy recommendations which are based solely on information on average cost calculations. Deviation from the average has as much relevance for costs as for clinical diagnoses and treatments.

Unless the organisation of care is so routinised or regimented – along the lines Goffman (1961) had in mind when he described the worst examples of ''total institutions'' – as to utterly disregard individual needs and circumstances, the costs of mental health services reflect patient or client differences. Thus, the clinician's concern with the presenting problems of individuals should be mirrored by an attempt to link costs to circumstances; indeed, the clinician's concern generates the need for this approach. However, service responses and the costs which summarise them are also shaped by, among other things, the preferences of other health and social care professionals working in the area, the bureaucratic tendencies of organisations, their scales of operation, and the characteristics of local economies and their implications for the supply of labour. Hence, the correspondence between the characteristics and costs of patients will not be unique. A host of intervening factors induces additional and perhaps counterbalancing variation, which the cost study must take into account. This can be done in one of two ways: (a) treat the 'extraneous' variation as 'noise' to be removed and disregarded, e.g. through the design of a randomised control trial (RCT) or by employing suitable techniques to 'partial them out' within a quasi-experimental design (with matched or statistical controls); or (b) explore these sources of cost variation so as to cast some light on the resource implications of practice and policy proposals. (Option (b) can be selected within a randomised or quasi-experimental design, although this is seldom done.) There are two reasons for preferring (b) to (a). Firstly, from the standpoint of policy – and all applied economists and most psychiatrists and other health and social care professionals should have an interest in policy – option (a) is singularly uninformative. Secondly, from the practice standpoint, an RCT helps us choose between alternative interventions with a degree of confidence which, in the right circumstances, cannot be approached by other evaluation methods. The quasi-experimental design is most often viewed as the second-best option. However, there are still few circumstances outside laboratory situations in which one can be sufficiently confident that all the assumptions necessary to validate an RCT hold true, and there are too many occasions on which the quasi-experimental design is employed only to remove 'contaminating influences'. The attractiveness of option (b) is that it provides additional insights without introducing additional assumptions.

The 'behavioural' cost function

In very few circumstances does the opportunity arise for an economic enquiry to be conducted under the kind of conditions which make an RCT possible. For this reason, a high proportion of applied economists have followed a multivariate approach, and in the study of costs, a large and impressive set of empirical examinations has now accumulated, based on the estimation of 'statistical cost functions'. The cost function follows directly from the economic theory of production, is based on assumptions which have been exhaustively debated in both market and non-market contexts, and has proved manageable and informative in application (Knapp, 1984, Ch. 9). If it is reasonable to make the analogy between, on the one hand, the production model of inputs and outputs and, on the other, the processes of delivering services to people with chronic mental illness, then the cost function approach has currency. It is, however, a data-hungry tool, a fact which limits its application, and in the wrong hands can be as dangerous and misleading as any other empirical procedure.

The cost function is most commonly estimated for a cross-sectional sample of 'production units' which are known or assumed to have reasonably similar objectives and to employ similar production techniques. In the study of manufacturing goods, the examination of the cost of production would ideally be based on data from a sample of factories (or work teams within factories) selling in the same market. We could then expect a statistically estimated representation of cost variation to reflect in part the underlying engineering processes which go to make up the production line. In service applications, there is no engineer's blueprint to guide the study of costs, and 'production' is certainly not routinised or standardised, but these circumstances need not invalidate the approach.

Much of economics is concerned with individual motivations and behaviour, and, in this respect, there is a great deal to borrow from psychology and other disciplines. The 'production unit' can therefore be defined at more than one level. Although data are more commonly available for higher aggregates, e.g. whole hospitals or residential care units, the cost and production functions which are readily employed and interpreted at those levels can also be used with more disaggregated data, such as those for individual users of mental health services. In a related service context, a 'production' theory has been developed to aid the analysis of individual well-being and its enhancement (Davies & Knapp, 1981). We spent some time examining the philosophical, psychological, and sociological literature on residential care for elderly people, using economic theories and metaphors to arrange them in the way which was (a) most likely to maximise the applicability of economic tools of analysis (of which the cost function is one), and (b) least likely to jettison the empirical insights that come from these other disciplines. The resultant ''production of welfare'' approach, as we termed it, has equal validity in other social and long-term care settings. Under the terms of this approach – and parallel theories in health economics generally – the cost function has a behavioural interpretation.

What does a cost function look like in practice? It is usually a multiple regression equation, with the dependent variable being either total cost (total amount expended) in a given time period (usually one financial year) or average cost (total cost divided by the number of people served or units of output produced). The explanatory or independent variables are suggested by a pragmatic blend of theory and experience in the field of inquiry, and are selected in any actual empirical study on these same criteria, plus statistical significance.

In this paper I shall use three cost functions estimated for mental health services in order to illustrate the costing rules set out above. One of those functions is presented immediately below; the other two follow later, and we shall therefore also be illustrating the need for the proper exploration and exploitation of cost variations.

Cost variations among hospitals

One of the controversial features of the present emphasis in the UK on running down the number of long-stay hospital beds is the way in which money is transferred from hospitals to 'the community'. The transfers are intended to facilitate the development of community provision, so that discharged hospital patients can move into a system of support services which is at least as good as hospital. Arrangements introduced in 1983 allow regional health authorities to make permanent transfers of money from hospital budgets to district health authority community mental health budgets, local authority social services departments, or voluntary organisations. These transfers out of hospital budgets – 'dowries' or 'bounties' – are tied to the permanent closure of hospital beds. They are usually based on some proportion of average hospital revenue cost, perhaps as much as 100%. The controversy sparked by these dowry transfers arises for a number of reasons. Hospital managers and consultant psychiatrists, among others, argue that money is being transferred out of their hospital budgets faster than it is being saved as beds close, because, *inter alia*, there are overhead costs which are not saved until whole wards or whole establishments close.

Using data for every psychiatric hospital in 10 of the 14 English health regions for each of three years, an average cost function was fitted in an attempt to estimate (after some differential calculus) the *marginal cost* of hospital in-patient care. The data were limited – e.g. no patient profiles or case mix information – but it was possible to make some progress towards an understanding of the average speed with which hospital costs fall as in-patient numbers decline. With one exception, previous UK studies of the costs of psychiatric hospital care do not permit a comparison with the results described below (Stern & Stern, 1963; Mercer, 1975; McKechnie *et al*, 1982). The exception is the unpublished doctoral dissertation of Casmas (1976), whose finding that average and marginal costs are similar in magnitude mirrors the finding from my study. I am not aware of any other European studies in this area, although there is some relevant US evidence, such as the work of Levenson *et al* (1977) in New York State.

Ordinary least squares estimation was used to fit a cost function, with average revenue cost per in-patient day as the dependent variable. (Out- and day-patient costs were omitted, as were all capital cost elements and any costs falling outside the hospital budget.) The independent or explanatory variables were the number of in-patient days, the proportion of available beds occupied over the year, and regional location (since regions have different policies for their long-stay hospital beds and face different labour supply prices). The 'best' representation of the cost function is detailed in Table 11.2, where 'best' refers to the conventional criteria of parsimony, statistical significance, and interpretability. From the function in the table, we can derive the marginal cost (by multiplication and then differentiation by the number of in-patient days), which, with the addition of regional effects, is equal to:

$$MC = 46.00 - 43.32 \times (\text{change in occupancy, 85/6 to 86/7})$$

Across all regions, and taking the mean change in occupancy across the 119 hospitals in the sample, marginal cost was £43 per in-patient day, or £298 per week, at 1986–87 prices. Yet the mean average cost per in-patient day for these same hospitals was £368. On average across the full sample, marginal cost – the cost of one additional or one fewer in-patient – was 81% of average revenue cost, and the estimated function indicates that this marginal cost will be higher in hospitals which are quicker to adjust their available beds to falling patient numbers. This is what should be expected: hospitals which have 'closed' beds (or whole wards or wings) as patients have moved out or died have smaller year-on-year changes in their occupancy

156   *Knapp*

TABLE 11.2
Statistical cost function for psychiatric hospitals, ten English regions, 1986–87

Variable	Coefficient	t-statistic
Inverse of number of in-patient days in 1986–87	104113	15.89***
Change in occupancy percentage, 1986–87 minus 1985–86	– 14.32	3.24***
Hospital located in Northern region	– 12.71	2.04**
Hospital located in Northwestern region	– 19.36	3.22***
Constant term	46.00	23.54***

Sample size = 119 $R = 0.72$ $F = 72.16$***

Dependent variable = average cost per in-patient day, 1986–87.
Significance: ***$P = 0.01$; **$P = 0.05$.

proportions, and therefore higher marginal savings. From this estimation exercise, therefore, we conclude that, on average, as much as 81% of a hospital's revenue cost is saved in the short term, as in-patient numbers decline; this is a much higher proportion than hospital managers claim they can save. They argue that overheads, such as management and centralised catering, which cannot be run down at the same speed as patient numbers, make it impossible for them to save very much in the short run. Certainly, the function assumes smooth cost adjustment, when the reality is a stepped process, but many hospitals are running down bed numbers at a speed that easily allows the annual closure of a whole ward, should this be professionally acceptable. However, financial transfers should not proceed at a pace which leaves hospitals denuded of resources, for this can quickly result in second-class settings for second-class patients (and staff).

It is not proposed that the 'dowry' transfers associated with hospital rundown should be governed by the results presented here, but estimates of this kind do provide a useful perspective on the financial implications for hospitals' moves towards long-term in-patient targets. They also offer evidence on economies of scale, which are pervasive, suggesting that the Victorians were clearly practising sound financial management when they built the huge asylums, although then, as today, patient welfare and other non-monetary considerations were at least as important in shaping services. These and other results which emerge from the exploration of cost variations must be used correctly. In one of his papers on the application of economic techniques to the evaluation of mental health services, Weisbrod (1983) made the point that cost-benefit analysis (or any applied tool of economics) cannot "*make* decisions", but it can "make decisions better informed".

Like-with-like comparisons

Once cost or other variations are reported, they invite comparisons. Why is one hospital more costly than another? Why does one group of patients impose a higher financial burden than another group? Why is mental health care more expensive in some parts of the country than others? These are important questions, and answers to them could well impinge on everything from national policy to the day-to-day decisions of individual clinicians. The problem is to avoid drawing the wrong conclusions because of misplaced comparisons, and the third costing rule says that only like-with-like comparisons give admissible evidence.

To explain and illustrate this third rule, consider the comparative costs of hospital and community care for people with chronic mental health problems in a period in which the former services are being run down to make way for the latter. It was the expected cost savings from a policy of community care which attracted the financial 'hawks' of government, and which put them in the unfamiliar position of supporting the professional preferences of many clinicians, nursing staff, and social workers. (The big difference between them was that these professional groups supported only a policy of *good* community care.) At first glance, community care seemed to offer considerable cost savings. The enthusiasm with which some people espoused a community care policy on cost grounds was exceeded only by their ignorance of the consequences of doing so. In the headlong pursuit of savings, nobody, it seemed, thought it necessary to test one of the fundamental assumptions on which the policy was based. Only in 1990 (in the UK at least, and this may also be true elsewhere in Europe) can we find evidence on the comparative costs (and patient outcomes) of hospital and community care which begins to meet the standards of scientific credibility.

The ideal evaluation of these comparative costs and outcomes would be a randomised control trial for the chronic care groups which are of interest. However, the word 'ideal' implies a stringent list of requirements, some of which are especially hard to meet when the policy background is the much-debated gradual run-down of hospital provision. Both politically and scientifically, it can be difficult to set up an RCT for this evaluation question. For the moment, we must interrogate evidence gathered within quasi-experimental designs with matched and/or statistical controls. The fundamental difference between the RCT and the quasi-experimental design in this context is that one leads clinical practice and the other follows it. The quasi-experimental design must examine what is already happening to patients whose destinations are determined not by the toss of a coin but by the decisions of professionals outside the research team. The cumulative effects of these past and present destination decisions in every country with which I am familiar is to leave the more 'dependent' or ill people in hospital, and to move or keep the less dependent or ill in the community. This makes a lot of political and professional sense, but it also makes it hard to evaluate the respective merits of the two settings.

It was noted earlier that hospital managers and staff have a number of problems with the UK policy of transferring money to 'the community' as long-stay beds close (even though this policy is in many respects a marked improvement on previous arrangements). Although community service managers have generally been more enthusiastic, they, too, have had some reservations about how the policy has worked in practice. The expectation is that the money previously spent on hospital in-patient services would all be transferred to fund community care; the dowry payment is the mechanism by which the money is shifted. Community managers have voiced the concern that dowries are insufficient to provide a decent standard of service, while hospital managers argue that dowries take more money from the hospital than is waranted by the need-generating characteristics of the patients who are moving. (This argument is distinct from concern about the speed with which transfers are made, which was considered above.) One group thus maintains that dowries are too small, and the other that they are too high, and both are probably correct. As a result, financial barriers are erected in front of community care (Knapp, 1990).

The problem is that the people moving from hospital to the community today are less dependent than the 'hospital average' or than those people who are not moving (Jones, 1989; Knapp *et al*, 1991, Ch. 5), yet they are more dependent, again comparing averages, than people in the same 'client group' already in the community. The errors that are often committed are to take today's costs of providing for today's clientele, and assume that the same amount of money will buy the same services (or achieve the same outcomes) for tomorrow's clientele. Given the common practice of moving less dependent in-patients to the community before more dependent patients, both hospital and community services can expect to experience some cost inflation, since the 'average degree of dependency' will increase in both settings, and with it the average cost. To test these arguments and to put some quantitative magnitudes on the likely future changes in costs, we can examine some early evidence emerging from an ongoing study of Friern and Claybury Hospitals in North London.

Cost predictions and extrapolations – illustrative evidence

As part of the research programme of the Team for the Assessment of Psychiatric Services (TAPS) directed by Julian Leff, information has been collected on all patients in Friern and Claybury Hospitals who meet certain research criteria (continuous hospital residence for at least a year and, if aged over 65, without a current diagnosis of dementia). The TAPS researchers are conducting a programme of linked evaluations from this baseline, particularly of the clinical outcomes of community reprovision for those people who move to the community (see Leff, this volume). The PSSRU is conducting linked economic evaluations of this reprovision programme.

One facet of the economic study relevant to this discussion of like-with-like comparisons is the examination of the association between the characteristics of individual hospital in-patients and the subsequent costs of their support in the community. If we then compare how the 'movers' from hospital compare with the 'stayers' we can make some predictions of community cost for the full eligible hospital populations. In this way, we can – for the first time in the UK – make informed guesses of the future cost of community care for comparison with the cost of hospital care (Knapp *et al*, 1990).

Community reprovision costs

By June 1989, a total of 146 people had left Claybury and 112 had left Friern under the region's hospital run-down plans; most were under the reprovision arrangements which carried dowry transfers, the first reprovision patients having moved to the community in 1985. Baseline information for all patients meeting the study criteria collected by TAPS ranged over a number of clinical dimensions, including mental health status, using the Present State Examination (PSE) and the Social Behaviour Schedule (SBS); the Physical Health Index (PHI); patient personal and historical data; patient attitudes; information on patients' social networks, using the Social Network Schedule (SNS); and an assessment of living environments. Altogether, including the 'new long-stay' patients who had accumulated in the two hospitals since the study began, baseline information had been assembled by TAPS on nearly 1000 patients.

The four previously described rules guided the costing of both hospital and community services. The costs of community care were based on retrospective accounts of service utilisation, accommodation descriptions and histories, staffing arrangements, and social security and other income receipts. They were defined so as to cover every service used, and priced so as to reflect long-run marginal costs of care, including the opportunity costs of capital. Thus, the costs for these first 'movers' are not artificially deflated just because the patients can be 'slotted into' existing residential, day-care, or other community facilities. The costing reflects service utilisation and living arrangements in the 12th month after leaving hospital, adjusted for regularly but infrequently used services such as occasional, short-term, in-patient stays over the full year in the community. The costs of psychiatric (community) reprovision are summarised in Table 11.3 for the first 145 leavers for whom data were collected. The mean cost per person per week, one year after leaving hospital, was £273, although varying by a factor of as much as 12 between the lowest- and highest-cost patients in the sample.

TABLE 11.3
The costs of psychiatric reprovision

Components of total cost	Percentage using the service %	Average weekly cost		% contribution to total %
		Users £	Full sample £	
Accommodation and living expenses	100	209	209	77.4
Hospital out-patient	21	9	2	0.7
Hospital day-patient	32	48	15	5.4
Other day care	38	33	12	4.5
Education services	10	33	3	1.2
Police	4	5	0	0.1
General practitioners	72	2	1	0.5
Injections	14	6	1	0.3
Nursing services	30	4	1	0.5
Psychiatrist	54	2	1	0.5
Social Worker	42	23	10	3.6
Miscellaneous professionals[1]	58	3	2	0.6
Travel	32	2	0	0.2
Volunteer inputs	4	17	1	0.3
Hospital in-patient stays	20	61	12	4.4

1. Chiropodist, optician, dentist, pharmacist, occupational therapist, physiotherapist, psychologist.
Total cost per person per week (1986–87 prices): average (mean), £270; standard deviation, £121; minimum, £47; maximum, £568.

The pattern of cost disaggregation is not dissimilar to that found for the Care in the Community demonstration programme sample (Table 11.1).

Cost predictions within the sample

The variation in community costs is to be explored in later analyses, in comparison to the outcome findings. The first research task was to examine the ability of the baseline (hospital) characteristics of leavers to explain observed variations in community costs. For this predictive purpose, only hospital-based information was accepted. Taking cost per week as the dependent variable and the full range of patient data collected by the TAPS interviews as the set of potential explanatory factors, ordinary least squares multiple regression was used to tease out the association. (Some of the potential explanatory variables are intercorrelated. This multicollinearity does not affect the overall predictive power of the equation or the validity of the extrapolations, but it does make it harder to disentangle the relative contributions of the variables. For this reason, we took a fairly generous cut-off level of significance ($P < 0.125$) in the analyses.)

The 'best' prediction equation, by the conventional criteria, is given in Table 11.4. The variable labels are explained in Table 11.5, which reports the basic statistical properties for these variables – for the sample of leavers

TABLE 11.4
The estimated reprovision cost prediction equation

Explanatory variables[1]	Coefficient	Significance[2]
Constant/intercept term	138.51	0.000
MALE	45.68	0.066
MALE × TOTNAM	− 3.28	0.007
LIFE	597.10	0.019
LIFE squared	− 968.54	0.024
STAY squared	0.002	0.016
STAY × AGE	− 0.10	0.067
STAY × TTMH	0.04	0.007
SBSTOT	11.56	0.003
PSENEG × AGE	0.75	0.006
PSENEG × TOTTIM	− 0.09	0.090

$R^2 = 0.355$ $R^2 = 0.300$ $F = 6.393$ (significance 0.000) $n = 127$

Dependent variable = cost per week at 1986–87 prices.
1. The variable labels are explained in Table 11.5.
2. Significance of t-test of individual coefficients.

TABLE 11.5
The hospital characteristics associated with reprovision cost

Variable		Sample of costed leavers			Full hospital populations		
		mean	s.d.	n	mean	s.d.	n
MALE	Indicator variable = 1 if male; 0 if female	0.52	0.50	136	0.57	0.50	964
AGE	Age at time of hospital assessment	54.96	14.22	136	58.24	15.98	963
STAY	Current length of stay (months)	154.78	171.04	136	222.09	211.90	964
TTMH	Total previous time in hospital (months)	52.99	89.10	136	42.64	78.44	964
TOTTIM	Total time ever in psychiatric hospital (months)	297.83	178.24	136	265.09	209.39	964
LIFE	Proportion of life spent in hospital	0.30	0.22	136	0.35	0.24	963
TOTNAM	Total number of named social contacts	11.61	9.33	120	8.68	6.94	604
SBSTOT	Score on Social behaviour Schedule (total)	3.44	2.90	136	5.50	3.44	963
PSENEG	Score on Present State Examination negative symptoms	1.02	1.08	133	1.25	1.27	951

for whom we had cost data and for all hospital residents meeting the study criteria. Overall, the equation explains 38% of the observed cost variation, which is a high level of statistical explanation, given the concentration on only baseline information. It implies that comprehensive hospital assessments of patients' needs can predict more than a third of the subsequent variation in community costs.

The equation in Table 11.4 offers some perspectives on those character-istics of hospital residents which are correlated with the subsequent needs for support in the community and hence with the costs of psychiatric reprovision. This is not the place to discuss these influences in detail; they are largely self-explanatory and are discussed elsewhere (Knapp, *et al*, 1990). However, the interpersonal variations in the costs of community care are certainly not random phenomena. They reflect, in part, the needs and other characteristics of patients. In this analysis, we find that patients' needs and characteristics in hospital have an effect on cost, through their bearing on community destinations and support needs, and because there is a correlation between characteristics in hospital and in the community. The second general point is that the cost predictors include a number of patient characteristics which distinguish the sample of movers from the full hospital population. The ramifications of this will become apparent in the extrapolations from these sample results to the full population. Thirdly, this is the first time that evidence beyond the anecdotal has been assembled on the cost-raising properties of in-patient characteristics.

Cost extrapolations to the full populations

Service planners need information not just on the costs of today's leavers, but accurate indications of the costs of supporting the whole hospital population once decanted, or that part of the population which will make the move. Only with such data can they begin to formulate long-term plans for community accommodation, day support, and peripatetic professional staff, as well as entering into informed discussions with other agencies about the coordination and subsidisation of policies and services.

Every time a costing is produced for former long-stay hospital patients now in the community, the riposte is heard that future hospital leavers will cost a lot more; this is based on one or more assumptions which we could reformulate as hypotheses. One assumption is that the first leavers from hospital are intrinsically less dependent and exhibit fewer symptoms of mental illness than those who remain behind to move in later cohorts, and this carries through to have a cost difference. This is the hypothesis we are testing here. Secondly, new capital projects are often not needed for the first leavers, because existing day and residential facilities can accommodate them, but substantial investment will be needed for future cohorts. This second assertion has validity in terms of flows of expenditure, but not in terms of costs, which are defined (as here) in terms of long-run marginal costs. A third but less common argument is that the supply price of certain types or grades of staff may rise with the growth of demand for them in the community. For example, a nationwide policy of psychiatric community reprovision generates a greater demand for community psychiatric nurses and social work staff. This third hypothesis is testable within a study of professional labour markets, but we cannot build the test into the present cost predictions, and its effects may be slight.

Employing the cost-prediction equation, we can extrapolate to the full populations of long-stay, non-demented in-patients in Claybury and Friern. For the extrapolations to be valid, in the sense that they are likely to give sensible predictions of future costs, the following conditions should hold: (a) the prediction equation must be robust (it is); (b) the sample for which the equation is estimated needs to be large enough to give confidence that the equation has some generalisability (it is, relative to the hospital populations); (c) the range of characteristics of the sample on the factors significantly associated with costs needs to be broad enough to overlap quite considerably with the range of characteristics of the remaining population (we believe it does, even though the first cohorts of leavers in general are comparatively less dependent and display fewer symptoms of psychiatric illness); and (d) missing values on cost-raising variables which arise because of the differential characteristics of the sample and population, such as self-reported descriptors which will not be available for those people unable to communicate, need to be handled with care, in order that they do not bias the extrapolations. (This has been done in this case with the variable measuring each patient's reported number of named social contacts, the only variable for which there were more than a small number of missing values.)

The results of the extrapolations are summarised in Table 11.6. The predicted reprovision costs for the 'stayers' – i.e. those patients who had not moved from hospital in time to be included in the cost equation analyses but who, under current plans, will move from hospital by the mid-1990s – cost approximately £61 more per week than the current average of £270 for all leavers to date.

Comparing hospital costs and predicted community costs

The predicted average community cost is thus £321 (per patient week, 1986–87 prices) for the full hospital populations. This is 19% above the reprovision costs measured for the sample of leavers. This predicted community cost is, however, less than the cost of hospital in-patient care in each of the two hospitals, including all relevant capital and indirect costs, at the time the reprovision programme commenced, in the hospital calculations. If we adjust hospital costs for the fact that patients with acute psychiatric illness or dementia are included in this hospital cost average, but are not part of the reprovision plans, and that these patients tend to receive more staff support and other services, we still find that future community costs are noticeably lower than the in-patient costs in Friern Hospital and marginally lower than in Claybury. This adjustment is based on a previous ward-costing exercise for Friern Hospital

TABLE 11.6
Cost predictions and extrapolations

Sample or population		Average cost per week: £ (1986–87 prices)				
		mean	s.d.	min.	max.	n
Costed leavers	– actual cost	270	121	47	568	136
	– predicted cost	269	77	39	505	133
All leavers	– predicted cost[1]	268	73	39	505	161
Stayers	– predicted cost[1]	332	88	119	882	789
Population	– predicted cost[1]	321	89	39	882	950

1. Predicted cost differs from actual because cost prediction is based on assumption that TOTNAM set equal to male population mean value of 8.66 for those males for whom this information is missing.

reported by Knapp *et al* (1987), which suggested that the first year's leavers from the hospital came from wards which cost 81% of the overall hospital average.

With this small difference between the costs of hospital in-patient care and the reprovision services, we may reject a commonly posited hypothesis about community care. The replacement of hospital with community services does not require the injection of substantial additional sums of money if patient quality of life is to be at least maintained and preferably improved. (The TAPS evaluation of the reprovision programme to date shows that patient welfare for the leavers is no worse than, and in some respects better than, that for the matched hospital sample.) The full costs of community provision can be met from hospital savings. Yet these outcome findings also imply that community care is not being provided 'on the cheap'. In these circumstances, the replacement of long-stay hospital residence with community reprovision of at least equivalent quality does not present any particular funding problems. However, there are potentially problems with, *inter alia*, the speed with which resources are transferred between the settings and the distribution of the cost burden in the community in comparison with the disbursements.

Merging costs and outcomes

It has been argued in this paper that it can be dangerous to discuss costs in isolation from outcomes. It is the merging of information on the two (the ideal) or recognition of the omission of one of them when drawing conclusions from analysis of the other (the pragmatic) which is the fourth rule of costing. The integration of costs and outcomes follows directly from the other three rules, and the discussion in the preceding three sections has taken us to a situation where it would be illogical not to look at them together. Among the likely sources of cost variation are patient characteristics and changes therein. Comparisons of like with like make it imperative for costs to be examined in the light of the outcomes that are achieved for patients and also for certain other people (such as relatives or neighbours). Costs and outcomes are inextricably linked – two parts of the same ('production') system. They are the inputs and outputs, means and ends, causes and effects, and it would be perverse to focus on one to the neglect of the other.

Because there is another paper in this volume on cost-effectiveness analysis, and because of the general drift of argument in this paper, this section does not attempt a comprehensive review of the evidence which combines costs with outcomes. Instead, the way that costs and outcomes can be jointly analysed will be illustrated, following the same methodological route as before.

The outcomes of the 'Care in the Community' programme

Above, the PSSRU's evaluation of the Care in the Community demonstration programme was introduced, and Table 11.1 reported some of the cost findings for the eight demonstration projects serving the (non-elderly) psychiatric client group. The community services delivered to these clients, when comprehensively costed, were less expensive than hospital care, even after adjustment for the fact that the people who moved were not representative of the full hospital population. This immediately prompts the question as to whether community care was being provided 'on the cheap', and whether it left clients with a lower quality of life than in hospital. The costings of the community care packages also showed much variation between clients (though not as marked as for the clients in the Friern and Claybury study reported above). Therefore, the questions need to be asked: does the cost variation reflect different client outcomes? Were more expensive care programmes also more successful in improving or maintaining the welfare of clients?

The general findings with regard to the outcomes of the demonstration programme are only briefly reported here, so as to preface the examination of their association with costs. (For a full account, see Knapp *et al*, 1991, Ch. 14) The client outcome findings for the Care in the Community programme were generally encouraging, and – interestingly – similar in many respects to the first evaluative findings reported from the TAPS evaluation of Friern and Claybury Hospitals. At the very least, the demonstration projects cannot be criticised for failing to ensure a satisfactory standard of care and support in the community for former hospital residents. The supposed 'failures' of hospital decanting policies were not evident in this programme. (No doubt they can be very real problems elsewhere, perhaps in less well-resourced and less well-planned situations, although one of the key purposes of the evaluation was to identify those factors and circumstances which are associated with 'successful' community care and which are replicable in the wider context.) In the Care in the

Community programme nobody was 'dumped' to drift without support, nobody was destitute or homeless, and nobody was imprisoned. There were few readmissions to hospital, and those that occurred were mainly of short duration and often for reasons unconnected to mental ill-health. Mortality rates were low, and the suicide rate less than 1% in the first nine months after discharge from hospital. The burden on 'informal carers' was very small, for the sad reason, perhaps, that few clients had informal care settings to which they could move. (The median length of continuous stay in hospital prior to the move was over 12 years, and most clients had either lost contact with relatives, or had relatives who were unable to make significant contributions to their care.) The impact on the wider community was evaluated only informally, although no pervasive evidence of unreasonable adverse effects could be found, except the danger (to community and clients alike) of 'ghettos' of former hospital patients building up in those areas with properties most suited to conversion to small-group living accommodation.

The central part of the evaluation was concerned with the welfare of clients, assessed along a number of dimensions both in hospital and in the community, approximately nine months after the move. The dimensions were: morale and life satisfaction, skills, behaviour, choice and empower-ment, personal presentation, activities and engagement, and social con-tacts and integration. (The measures used are described below; not all of them lend themselves to quantitative analysis.) Integration into community lifestyles and 'ordinary' settings was far from complete, but most clients were using 'ordinary' services such as shops, pubs, GPs, or churches, and there was much more activity outside the confines of the place of residence than these people had enjoyed when they had been living in hospital. Twice as many patients expressed positive attitudes about activities in the community, compared to their preferences in hospital. Most of them had more choice about how they spent their time and the activities they engaged in, although more generous social security benefits or the availability of 'real' employment would extend the range of choice closer to the breadth enjoyed by most citizens. Although it takes time for people to build up social networks, reported social contacts were greater in number in the community than in hospital. Skill levels and behavioural problems and symptoms (as reported by staff) were no different between hospital and community, although there were some slight differences between the different types of community settings to which people moved. Self-report measures of satisfaction with the environment, psychosocial functioning, depression, satisfaction with social interaction, and global morale revealed borderline improvements between hospital and community (attaining significance at the 5% level).

Overall, the evaluation of client outcomes suggested that there was no reason to believe that community living within the demonstration programme is going wrong: negative outcomes had been avoided and client quality of life was generally no worse than in hospital. There were, however, relatively few observed improvements in quality of life in the first nine months after leaving hospital.

Community and hospital comparisons

It should be noted that the simple comparisons of hospital and community welfare and costs for the group of leavers reveal that: (a) community care is noticeably less costly than hospital for this cohort; and (b) community care is at least as good as hospital in maintaining standards of client welfare. This result is thus in line with the North East Thames study findings already mentioned, and consistent with the US results of Cassel *et al* (1972), Murphy & Datel (1976), and Weisbrod *et al* (1980), although these are concerned with different policy contexts. It was also found, not surprisingly, that the most dependent clients received packages of services which were more costly than hospital, again consistent with our NETRHA findings (see Table 11.6 for evidence) and with Häfner & an der Heiden (1989).

Costs, client characteristics, and outcomes

It is reasonable to hypothesise that the costs of the packages of community care services received by individual clients will vary in response to, or be associated with, differences in levels of need and changes in need, the latter measuring the principal outcomes of an intervention. With the accumulation of experience on the needs and preferences of chronically mentally ill people living outside hospital, with the growing emphasis on efficiency in the utilisation of resources, and with the increasing coordination of services through case management and similar procedures, there are good reasons for expecting strong associations between costs, client characteristics, and outcomes. (These associations will be mediated through such other factors as scale and organisation of service delivery agencies, organisational style, regional location and its effects on the prices of inputs, etc., each of which is of interest in its own right.) These hypotheses were tested through the estimation of a series of cost functions. In contrast to the empirical work reported in Table 11.4, these functions focus on the characteristics of clients in the community, as well as on changes in these characteristics since the assessments in hospital.

Client characteristics for which there were quantitative measures for exploration in relation to cost differences were: *skills level*, a measure of adaptive behaviour developed for the evaluation of the multiple client group from other instruments (see Renshaw *et al*, 1988, Ch. 11); *behavioural problems* and symptoms, or maladaptive behaviour, again based on purpose-built instrumentation; *level of and satisfaction with social interaction*, using the Schedule for Social Interaction (Henderson, 1981); *depression* measured by the

Depression Inventory of Snaith *et al* (1971); *morale*, taken from the morale subscale of the Psychosocial Functioning Inventory of Feragne *et al* (1983) and the 'ladder' of life satisfaction developed by Cantrill (1965); and *personal presentation*, as rated by interviewers using a short instrument developed in the PSSRU. Scores on these instruments were recorded both in hospital (usually prior to a patient's participation in a hospital-based rehabilitation programme, and sometimes some months before discharge to the community) and in the community approximately nine months after the move. We thus had both 'absolute' and 'relative' (change) measures of client welfare or needs.

These client-specific measures were used as predictors of cost differences in the cost-function analyses, along with measures of various mediating factors. The analyses were complicated by the fact that some background information was not available for all clients, and because there are different sets of potential mediating factors which can be included in different ways. It is therefore necessary to look at more than one series of estimates in order to draw conclusions about cost-outcome associations. The regression equations are not reported here, but are detailed in Knapp *et al* (1991, Ch. 14) and in Knapp & Beecham (1990). Table 11.7 provides a summary of the results from six separate series of analyses.

Community care costs are clearly sensitive to most of the client features for which measures were developed. Costs are higher for people displaying greater needs along the dimensions spanned by the skills scale, the rating of behavioural problems and symptoms, the Schedule for Social Interaction, Cantrill's ladder of life satisfaction, and the rating of personal presentation. On each instrument, a lower score indicates lower quality of life or more 'problems', and the negative relationship between these scores and costs is an indication of the responsiveness of care resources and agencies to the health and social welfare needs of clients. This is what one would hope to observe from an integrated and carefully planned system of care services, but England does not have such a system, and the consistency must be attributable in large measure to the case management practices which were adopted, and which were, in fact, a condition for the funding of demonstration projects. One dimension of client welfare deviates from this general finding: higher scores on the morale subscale of the Psychosocial Functioning Inventory are associated with higher costs, which is interpreted as a causal linkage running from service utilisation to contentment.

Changes in client characteristics play only a small role in the explanation of cost variations. Both absolute and relative differences in well-being scores were examined, but the effects are small, even though statistical significance was achieved after standardising for differences in client background circumstances, hospital-based assessments of need, and some organisational features of the different demonstration projects. Higher costs are associated with the attainment of greater or better outcomes in relation to behavioural

TABLE 11.7
Summary of care in the community cost function results

Variable	Significance	Range[2]
Age at T1	+ ve	0.000–0.004
Duration of hospital stay before discharge[1]	– ve	0.000–0.032
Original diagnosis: organic brain disorder	+ ve	0.001–0.053
Age at onset of mental illness	– ve	0.001
Skills score at T2	– ve	0.017
Behavioural problems score at T2[1]	– ve	0.000–0.141
Schedule for Social Interaction at T2	– ve	0.015–0.034
Psychosocial Functioning Inventory at T2	+ ve	0.029–0.106
Cantrill morale score at T2	– ve	0.025–0.114
Personal presentation score at T2	– ve	0.001–0.054
Behaviour change: (T2–T1) or (T2–T1/T1)	+ ve	0.000–0.015
Cantrill change: (T2–T1)	+ ve	0.001
Personal presentation change: (T2–T1)	+ ve	0.186
Depression Inventory change: (T2–T1)	+ ve	0.003–0.039
Client readmitted to hospital[3]	+ ve	0.018–0.086
Size of community accommodation (no. places)	+ ve	0.001
Case management delegated to keyworker	– ve	0.017–0.064
Clients involved in case management	+ ve	0.000
Project management at strategic not local level	– ve	0.005

T1 = hospital assessment; T2 = community assessment.
1. Variable appears in non-linear form.
2. Range of significance of *t*-tests in the 'best' equations coming from each cost function series. In some equations variables did not enter the 'best' functions, or were excluded on the basis of *a priori* restrictions (see Knapp & Beecham, 1990).
3. Two variables (incidence and duration) were employed in the analyses with mixed effects, generally indicating that post-discharge in-patient stays push up costs.

problems, symptoms, morale, personal presentation, and depression. The effects are again as would be expected on the basis of deductive reasoning or anecdote, though not on the basis of previous research, because there appears to be little evidence to confirm or deny such suppositions. It is interesting, therefore, that although improvements in the welfare of clients were modest at an aggregate level, once we delve into interclient variations we uncover significant positive associations with cost.

These examinations reveal that higher community care costs are not only attributable to higher levels of observed need in the community, but are also associated with greater achievements in reducing this need. We can conclude that higher levels of spending on community care will generate further improvements in quality of life. Whether the additional expenditure is warranted by the welfare improvements cannot, however, be examined here.

Other influences on cost

To the majority of mental health care evaluators, it is the link between costs and outcomes which is of primary interest, but other factors have an influence and a relevance for policy. In the mode of the RCT, these are the contaminating factors whose influences must be removed by randomisation, whereas in the mode of the quasi-experimental design, they are removed by some combination of matching and statistical analysis. They are, however, of more than passing interest in their own right. Häfner & an der Heiden (1989) have argued that "studies should look for clearly definable components of the complex package of care to determine whether they are effective, and for which diagnostic categories of patients" (p. 60). The same must also apply to the examination of costs.

A small number of indicator ('dummy' or 'zero-one') variables describing organisational characteristics of the demonstration projects and their case management arrangements were introduced into some of the cost function explorations. The results are summarised in Table 11.7, and suggest some influence on costs. Strategic (area level) rather than localised planning appears to be associated with lower costs, other things being equal, and consumer involvement in decision-making appears to be associated with higher costs. The small number of different service systems covered by this analysis should induce caution against hurried generalisations from these two findings. The same is not the case for a further set of potential cost-raising factors examined in this study – each client's accommodation 'type' in the community.

The package of services received by a client is tailored to some extent by individual needs and circumstances. However, for the purposes of discussion and planning, some typology of community arrangements which cuts through this individual variability is often needed. The most common basis for such a typology is residential accommodation, even though it is widely recognised that places of residence cannot or ought not meet the full range of needs of people with chronic psychiatric illness. Thus, planning statements are couched in terms of, e.g., 'more hostel facilities', or 'more people in unstaffed group homes'. A key policy question, then, is whether and how the costs of complete community care packages vary between accommodation types. This question was examined by testing for a statistical association between the residual (unexplained) costs from the cost functions and the types of accommodation occupied by clients. Seven accommodation types were represented in the demonstration projects: residential care homes (11 clients for whom we had cost data), hostels (52), staffed group homes (13), unstaffed group homes (40), foster homes (5), supported lodgings (3), and independent living (6). Each accommodation label was attached by the research team on the basis of consistently applied criteria. The analyses revealed few significant associations between costs and accommodation type; tentatively, it was concluded that residential care homes and staffed group homes are more expensive than other settings, having standardised for differences in client characteristics and outcomes, and that independent living arrangements are less expensive.

Conclusion

In this paper I have looked at four principal topics: (a) the policy and political contexts in which demands arise for cost information; (b) the nature and phasing of those demands; (c) four basic rules to guide the empirical costs research which can most usefully meet demands; and (d) concomitant implications for the design, execution, and interpretation of their research. Changes in mental health care policy or practice which ignore costs, or which embody cost information without obeying or recognising the four basic rules, can be of only dubious validity, or can be used to answer only a limited range of questions. But, as the illustrative studies have shown, it need not be a horrendous, or ideologically compromising, or scientifically complex task to add a cost dimension to the evaluation of mental health services. There are enough examples in the literature of bad costs research to demonstrate that it is not as simple as some have thought, but there are also enough examples of good research to encourage further attempts.

Acknowledgement

This paper draws partly on research funded by the UK Department of Health and the North East Thames Regional Health Authority, and conducted jointly with colleagues in the Personal Social Services Research Unit, University of Kent at Canterbury, particularly Jeni Beecham, Paul Cambridge, Corinne Thomason, and Caroline Allen. Some of the material reported here comes from an ongoing collaborative study with the Team for the Assessment of Pscyhiatric Services led by Julian Leff. The paper was written while I was a visiting International Fellow in the Institute for Policy Studies, Johns Hopkins University, Baltimore. I extend my gratitude to all these for their assistance, but absolve them from all responsibility for the views expressed in this paper. A shorter version of this paper was published in *Psychological Medicine*, 1990.

References

CANTRILL, H. (1965) *The Pattern of Human Concerns*. New Brunswick, NJ: Rutgers University Press.

CASMAS, S. T. (1976) *Inter-hospital and Inter-local Authority Variation in Patterns of Provision for the Mentally Disordered*. PhD thesis, University of Manchester Institute of Science and Technology.

CASSEL, W. A., SMITH, C. M., GRUNBERG, F., *et al* (1972) Comparing costs of hospital and community care. *Hospital and Community Psychiatry*, **23**, 197–200.

CONLEY, R. W., CONWELL, M. & ARRILL, M. B. (1973) An approach to measuring the cost of mental illness. *American Journal of Psychiatry*, **124**, 755–762.

DAVIES, B. & KNAPP, M. (1981) *Old People's Homes and the Production of Welfare*. London: Routledge and Kegan Paul.

DICKEY, B., CANNON, N., McGUIRE, T., *et al* (1986) The quarterway house: a two-year cost study of an experimental residential program. *Hospital and Community Psychiatry*, **37**, 1136–1143.

FEIN, R. (1958) *The Economics of Mental Illness*. New York: Basic Books.

FERAGNE, M. A., LONGABAUGH, R. & STEVENSON, J. F. (1983) The Psychosocial Functioning Inventory. *Evaluation and the Health Professions*, **6**, 25–48.

GINSBERG, G. & MARKS, I. (1977) Costs and benefits of behavioural psychotherapy: a pilot study of neurotics treated by nurse-therapists. *Psychological Medicine*, **7**, 685–700.

GOFFMAN, E. (1961) *Asylums: Essays on the Social Situation of Mental Patients and Other Inmates*. Harmondsworth: Penguin.

HÄFNER, H. & AN DER HEIDEN, W. (1989) Effectiveness and cost of community care for schizophrenic patients. *Hospital and Community Psychiatry*, **40**, 59–63.

HENDERSON, S. (1981) *Neurosis and the Social Environment*. Sydney: Academic Press.

HURST, J. (1988) Report of a meeting held in July 1987 at the Institute of Psychiatry. In *New Directions in Mental Health Care Evaluation*, (eds I. Marks, J. Connelly and M. Muijen). London: Institute of Psychiatry.

JONES, D. (1989) Unpublished paper from the Team for the Assessment of Psychiatric Services. London: Friern Hospital.

——, GOLDBERG, D. & HUGHES, B. (1980) A comparison of two different services treating schizophrenia: a cost-benefit approach. *Psychological Medicine*, **10**, 493–505.

KNAPP, M. (1984) *The Economics of Social Care*. London: Macmillan.

—— (1990) Economic barriers to innovation in mental health care: community care in the UK. In *Innovation in Mental Health Care Delivery*, (eds I. Marks & R. Scott). London: Cambridge University Press.

——, RENSHAW, J. & BEECHAM, J. (1987) The cost-effectiveness of psychiatric reprovision services: an interim report. Discussion Paper 533, Personal Social Services Research Unit, University of Kent at Canterbury.

——, BEECHAM, J., *et al* (1990) Predicting the community costs of closing psychiatric hospitals. *British Journal of Psychiatry*, **157**, 661–670.

—— & —— (1990) The cost-effectiveness of community care for former long-stay psychiatric hospital patients. Discussion Paper 628, Personal Social Services Research Unit, University of Kent at Canterbury (Available from the authors).

——, CAMBRIDGE, P., THOMASON, C., *et al* (1991) *Care in the Community: Challenge and Demonstration*. Aldershot: Gower.

LEVENSON, A. J., LORD, C. J. & SERMAN, C. E. (1977) Acute schizophrenia: an efficacious treatment approach as an alternative to full-time hospitalisation. *Diseases of the Nervous System*, **38**, 242–245.

MCKECHNIE, A. A., RAE, D. & MAY, J. (1982) A comparison of in-patient costs of treatment and care in a Scottish psychiatric hospital. *British Journal of Psychiatry*, **140**, 602–607.

MANGEN, S. P., PAYKEL, E. S., GRIFFITH, J. H., *et al* (1983) Cost-effectiveness of community psychiatric nurse or out-patient psychiatrist care of neurotic patients. *Psychological Medicine*, **13**, 407–416.

MARKS, I., CONNOLLY, J. & MUIJEN, M. (1988) The Maudsley Daily Living Programme: a controlled cost-effectiveness study of community based versus standard in-patient care of serious mental illness. *Bulletin of the Royal College of Psychiatrists*, **12**, (January), 22–23.

MERCER, A. D. (1975) A model for nursing cost. *Hospital and Health Services Review*, **71**, 194–195.

MURPHY, J. G. & DATEL, W. E. (1976) A cost-benefit analysis of community versus institutional living. *Hospital and Community Psychiatry*, **27**, 165–170.

RENSHAW, J., HAMPSON, R., THOMASON, C., *et al* (1988) *Care in the Community: the First Steps*. Aldershot: Gower.

SNAITH, R. P., AHMED, S. N., MEHTA, S., *et al* (1971) Assessment of the severity of primary depressive illness. *Psychological Medicine*, **1**, 143–149.

STERN, B. & STERN, E. S. (1963) Efficiency of mental hospitals. *British Journal of Preventive and Social Medicine*, **17**, 111–120.

THOMASON, C. & BEECHAM, J. (1988) Supporting people with long-term needs in the community. In *Social Security and Community Care*, (eds S. Baldwin, G. Parker & R. Walker). Aldershot: Avebury.

WEISBROD, B. A. (1983) A guide to benefit-cost analysis, as seen through a controlled experiment in treating the mentally ill. *Journal of Health Politics and Law*, **7**, 809–845.
———, TEST, M. A. & STEIN, L. I. (1980) Alternative to mental hospital treatment: economic benefit-cost analysis. *Archives of General Psychiatry*, **37**, 400–405.

12 Cost-effectiveness of community care for the chronic mentally ill

OWEN O'DONNELL

The resources available for improving or maintaining the quality of life of the chronic mentally ill are scarce, but this is no different from all of life's activities. Resources are scarce in whatever we have to do, and the logical consequence of this universal scarcity is choice. Choice involves sacrifice: in choosing to do one thing, we are sacrificing the benefits of doing other things – everything has an opportunity cost. To devote more resources to health care means sacrificing the benefits to be received from other public services, such as education. To devote more resources to meet the objectives of better mental health means sacrificing more health care for other people. Allocating more resources to the care of individuals with a chronic mental health problem deprives others with an acute mental illness of services. It is because these sacrifices are incurred that the resources allocated to the care of the chronic mentally ill are limited.

There are a number of ways of using these scarce resources to improve the quality of life of individuals with a chronic mental health problem, e.g. in-patient care, day hospitals, out-patient clinics, support in the community, employment training, and better housing. The costs of deploying resources in one programme are the benefits foregone from alternative uses. Maximising the quality of life of the chronic mentally ill requires allocating resources to those programmes which achieve the greatest benefit at a given cost or a given benefit at the least cost. In other words, the most efficient pro-grammes must be selected.

Economic evaluation provides a framework for making choices between competing uses of resources, by identifying the costs and benefits of those alternatives. The prerequisites for an evaluation are that an objective be defined and the alternative methods of achieving this identified. It will be assumed that the objective of maximising the quality of life of the chronic mentally ill commands widespread support. There appears to be little consensus on how this can be achieved. Many countries have adopted the policy of shifting care from institutions to the community. But there is a great deal of inter- and intra-country variation in the extent to which this policy has been implemented (Goldman *et al*, 1983). Evidence on the efficiency of care in the community, as an alternative to institutional care, is required to facilitate more informed decision-making. Furthermore, since community care can take a variety of forms, evaluation is required to identify the most efficient form for each type of individual.

The framework of economic evaluations

The identification of costs and benefits forms the basis of an economic evaluation. Efficiency is assessed from a societal perspective; it involves using society's resources to maximise its welfare. In evaluating a mental health care programme, the costs and benefits to all sectors of society are relevant: it is not sufficient to identify the costs to the direct providers of treatment. The costs of community care include resources provided by all public and private welfare services, voluntary organisations, clients, and their friends and relatives. Similarly, benefits can extend beyond those experienced by the recipients of treatment.

The primary benefits of care are improvements in the health and quality of life of the recipients and of their friends and relatives. These benefits have been measured along dimensions, such as symptom remission, role functioning, and self-esteem. Since these benefits are multidimensional and non-monetary, the net benefit (i.e. benefits minus costs) of a mental health care programme usually cannot be calculated. The efficiency of treatments must be compared by separate comparisons of costs and each dimension of outcomes. This approach is unproblematic when one alternative dominates costs and every outcome dimension, but when this is not the case, it is not possible to identify the most efficient alternative from the evaluation. This does not mean, however, that evaluation is useless in such circumstances. Since evaluation presents information on the costs and effectiveness of each alternative to decision-makers, they can assess whether the extra benefits of one treatment are worth the extra costs, or poorer outcomes along another dimension. In doing this, the decision-makers are forced to make their judgement about the value of the extra benefits explicit, and the public can hold them responsible for such judgements.

The relevant costs in an economic evaluation are given by opportunity costs, i.e. the benefit foregone from discarded options. These costs are not always monetary; for instance, time spent by friends and relatives caring for individuals with a chronic mental health problem can involve costs, in the form of foregone household production (e.g. housework, DIY) or leisure activities. The psychological and emotional burden of caring represents additional costs to informal carers. Opportunity costs are not synonymous with financial costs. Transfer payments do not represent a net cost to society; they are simply transfers of resources between members of society, and since efficiency is assessed from a societal perspective, transfer payments are not relevant to the assessment of costs. The concept of opportunity cost is also helpful in identifying the capital costs of a programme. As long as capital has an alternative use, there is a cost of continuing with its present use. For example, there is a capital cost of continuing to use a psychiatric hospital for the care of chronically ill patients, even after the land, buildings, and equipment have been paid for, as long as the hospital could be used in some other way. If the hospital could be sold, then the capital cost is its market value.

The evidence which currently exists on the efficiency of community care for individuals with a chronic mental health problem will be reviewed below, with the aim of assessing whether the evidence available is sufficient to plan an efficient programme of care in the community. The review begins with discussion of evaluations of alternative forms of hospital-based care. Attention is then given to the evidence on the efficiency of community care options, detached from psychiatric hospitals, as alternatives to hospital admission. Finally, the evidence on the efficiency of alternative types of care in the community is reviewed. For each section, a table is presented, in which the main features of the studies are described. The criteria for inclusion in the review are that the alternatives evaluated are relevant to the transition from institutional to community care of individuals with a chronic mental illness, and that both the costs and effectiveness of the alternatives have been evaluated. Additionally, only studies published in English are included: as a result, North American and UK studies predominate; the review cannot claim to be truly international.

Hospital-based alternatives

The most conservative step in the transition from institutional to community care has been to shift in-patient care from psychiatric hospitals to psychiatric units in general hospitals. Two studies, carried out by the same group in Manchester, evaluated the efficiency of in-patient care in a district general hospital, compared with an area mental hospital, for first-admission schizophrenic patients (Jones *et al*, 1980; Jones & Goldberg, 1980; see Table 12.1). In each study, the assessment of both monetary and non-monetary costs and benefits favoured the general hospital, but the design of these studies places the validity of results in some doubt. Rather than being prospective controlled trials, the appraisals were based on four- and 12-year retrospective follow-up studies of patients treated at each of the alternatives. Although no differences in the socio-demographic compositions of the cohorts were identified, there is no way of ensuring that the results reflect differences in the outcomes of the treatments received, rather than differences in the severity of the conditions experienced by patients treated in each setting.

TABLE 12.1
Hospital-based alternatives

Study	Experimental treatment (E)	Control treatment (C)	Type of patients	Type of study	Number in sample[1]	Enumeration		Costs	Results
						Outcomes			
Psychiatric versus general hospital									
Jones et al (1980) (UK)	In-patient stay in psychiatric unit of teaching district general hospital	In-patient stay in area mental hospital	First admission schizophrenics; exclusion criteria: brain damage, drug abuse, alcoholism, or epilepsy	4-year retrospective follow-up	E = 55 (81%) C = 51 (77%)	Diagnosis, symptoms, social performance attitudes, unmet need, earnings		Direct and indirect treatment costs to health and social services; burden on families	Clinical outcome similar; unmet need and family burden lower for E; net economic benefit favoured E
Jones & Goldberg (1980) (UK)	In-patient stay in psychiatric unit of district general hospital	In-patient stay in area mental hospital	First admission schizophrenics; exclusion criteria: brain damage, drug abuse, alcoholism, or epilepsy	12-year retrospective follow-up	E = 50 (67%) C = 49 (67%)[2]	Psychiatric state, psycho-social assessment, earnings		Direct and indirect treatment costs to health and social services; burden on families	E more effective and net economic benefit higher than C
Short versus long in-patient stay									
Glick et al (1974) (USA)	Brief in-patient stay (21–28 days)	Long in-patient (90–120 days)	Schizophrenic patient	Randomised controlled trial (RCT) 1-year follow-up	E = 31 (100%) C = 30 (100%)	Symptoms, psychiatric, social, work and family functioning; leisure activity; readmissions		Post-hospital treatment costs	C had higher global outcomes and less readmissions
In-patient versus out-patient									
Levenson et al (1977) (USA)	Daily visit to out-patient clinic	In-patient care	Acute schizophrenia; excluded those of harm to self or others	RCT, follow-up to remission or treatment transfer	E = 10 (100%) C = 10 (100%)	Symptoms, psychiatric state		Direct treatment and transport costs	No difference in outcomes; E cheaper

Continued

TABLE 12.1
Continued

Study	Experimental treatment (E)	Control treatment (C)	Type of patients	Type of study	Number in sample[1]	Enumeration		Results
						Outcomes	Costs	
Häfner & an der Heiden (1989) (FRG)	Out-patient care	None	Schizophrenics	Uncontrolled cohort study	148 (76%)	Symptoms, behaviour, hospitalisation	Direct cost to health and social services	Out-patient care negatively correlated with hospitalisations and positively with outcomes; average cost of out-patient 43% of in-patient
Day hospital versus in-patient								
Washburn et al (1976) (USA)	Brief in-patient followed by day hospital	In-patient care	Female, privately financed; functional disorder	RCT (18-month follow-up)	59 (100%) (36% of inital sample randomised)	Psychopathology, social adjustment, satisfaction	Private charges; family burden	E dominant on costs and outcomes
Endicott et al (1978) (USA)	Brief in-patient followed by day hospital and out-patient care or out-patient only	Long in-patient with discharge to out-patient care	Functional illness and in contact with family; excluding: organic brain disease, alcoholism, drug addiction, and antisocial personality	RCT (2 year follow-up)	E = 118 C = 63 (attrition not reported)	Psychopathology, role functioning	Direct costs to health services; financial and non-financial burden on families	E dominant on costs and outcomes

Study				Design	Sample	Outcomes	Costs	Conclusions
Dick *et al* (1985) (UK)	Day hospital	In-patient care	Emergency admissions; diagnoses of neuroses, adjustment reaction or personality disorder (exclusion criteria reported elsewhere)	RCT (4-month and 1-year follow-up)	E = 38 (88%)[3] C = 45 (94%) (27% of relevant admissions randomised)	Psychiatric state, work status, patient satisfaction	Direct and indirect costs to health and social services; travel and subsistence costs	No difference in outcomes; E 65% of cost of cheapest in-patient care
Hospital versus hostel ward								
Wykes (1982) (UK)	Hostel ward on the site of a psychiatric hospital	Ward of psychiatric or general hospital	'New long-stay' 18–65 years; no organic brain disease	Before and after study	E = 13 (100%) C = 12 (100%)	Social performance, time budgets, patient attitudes, quality of care	Revenue costs to health service only	Hostel more effective; hostel cheaper then general hospital but more expensive than psychiatric hospital
Hyde *et al* (1987) (UK)	Hostel ward on the site of a psychiatric hospital	Ward in psychiatric unit of general hospital	Length of stay ⩾ 6 months; need of 24-hour nursing care; no serious harm to self or public	Matched pairs with random allocation (2-year follow-up)	E = 11 (100%) C = 11 (100%)	Problem behaviour and impairments, clinical state, social behaviour, satisfaction	Direct and indirect costs to health and social services; law enforcement costs; capital costs	E dominant on costs and outcomes

1. Figures refer to the number who completed follow-up and, in parentheses, the percentage of the initial sample.
2. Excludes those dead or emigrated at follow-up.
3. Figures give numbers completing four-month follow-up.

G

A further feature of the transition towards community care has been the replacement of continuous in-patient care with brief periods of hospital admission. Glick *et al* (1974; see Table 12.1) evaluated short-term (21–28 days) versus long-term (90–120 days) in-patient treatment for schizophrenic patients. Although the study was based on a randomised controlled trial (RCT), a disproportionate number of both non-white patients and patients from lower socio-economic groups were allocated to the short-term group. This may partly explain the relatively poorer performance of this group on global outcome and readmission rates. Also, the costing component of this study was rather illogical: only post-hospital treatments were costed. No significant differences between the groups in these costs were reported; this result is consistent with higher total costs of long-term in-patient care.

The fact that the outcomes of the long-term group were slightly superior may reflect the fact that brief hospital admission was not accompanied by an after-care programme. This leaves the possibility that brief hospital admission followed by a programme of out-patient visits or day care could provide an efficient alternative to long periods of in-patient care. The relative efficiency of out-patient versus in-patient care has been examined by Levenson *et al* (1977; see Table 12.1). Patients with acute schizophrenia were randomly allocated either to daily visits to an out-patient clinic or to in-patient care. There were only ten patients in each group – a sample size too small to test the hypothesis that out-patient treatment is more efficient than in-patient care. The average cost of in-patient care per remission was found to be six times that of out-patient care, but it is likely that the magnitude of this cost difference reflects the narrow costing carried out, rather than the true difference in societal resources consumed by each alternative. The only services costed were those provided by the hospital and out-patient clinic, plus the costs of transport to the clinic; costs to social services and informal carers were excluded, and these omissions bias the cost comparison in favour of the community care alternative.

A more recent study (Häfner & an der Heiden, 1989; see Table 12.1) attempted to measure the efficiency of out-patient care for schizophrenic patients, using an alternative to the conventional method of comparing two groups of patients allocated to treatment alternatives. The approach taken involved fitting multiple regression models in order to predict use of out-patient care over 12 months, and outcomes, measured by symptoms and illness-related behaviour, over the subsequent six months. The independent variables in each model were psychopathology, living situations, and chronicity of illness. The correlations between the residuals of observed minus expected out-patient care and outcomes were then examined. Greater-than-average (predicted) use of out-patient care was found to be correlated with better-than-average (predicted) outcomes and lower use of in-patient treatment in the subsequent six months. The validity of this method is dependent upon the specification of the models of both out-patient care and outcomes. Any under- or mis-specifications could produce spurious correlations between the quantity of out-patient care and outcomes. In view of this potential for error, the presentation of the results is weakened by the fact that no information is given on the fit of any of the models.

The logic of the comparison of costs in the analysis is not obvious. The average cost of community care was found to be 43% of the cost of continuous care in hospital, but it is reported that only three out of a total of 148 patients in the cohort experienced continuous hospital care. For the majority of patients, continuous in-patient care does not appear to be a relevant alternative. Furthermore, the study examined the effectiveness of greater-than-average (predicted) out-patient care. The relevant cost comparison, therefore, is not given by the average cost (i.e. total costs divided by total treatments) of out-patient and in-patient care, but by the costs of additional out-patient care, which should be compared with the additional benefits generated. Additional costs are known as marginal costs: these, rather than average costs, are relevant whenever it is a change in the size of a service which is being evaluated. There are a number of reasons why marginal costs may differ from average costs. Firstly, average costs do not allow for the intensity with which resources are currently being used. For example, if a hostel in the community has spare capacity, the additional cost of caring for more patients in that hostel would be small, since the resources already available can be used more intensively; using average costs would overestimate the costs of raising the level of activity, since this would assume there was no spare capacity. Secondly, it is likely that costs will be related to the characteristics of the patients treated. Häfner & an der Heiden (1989) acknowledged this, pointing out that the difference between the average costs of in-patient and community care overestimates the savings to be made from discharging patients, since community care costs will rise as patients with more severe disturbances are discharged.

Day hospitals provide another alternative to full-time hospital care. Three RCTs have examined the cost-effectiveness of day hospitals, relative to in-patient care. Two of these evaluated care for patients with functional disorders (Washburn *et al*, 1976; Endicott *et al*, 1978; see Table 12.1); the third focused on patients with a diagnosis of neurosis, adjustment reaction, or personality disorder (Dick *et al*, 1985; see Table 12.1). In the former two studies, carried out, respectively, in Massachusetts and New York, patients experienced a brief in-patient stay, followed by either continued hospital care or discharge to day hospital or out-patient care. Both of the studies were limited to particular types of patients: Washburn *et al* (1976) included only female patients who could finance their own care, and Endicott *et al* (1978) included only patients in contact with their families. Whether the results generalise to patients without these characteristics is not known.

The costing employed in each of these studies was rather crude. In the Massachusetts study, the only costs identified were charges for medical care made to the patients, while in the evaluation carried out in New York, the average cost figures employed were not specific to the facilities actually used by the patients in the study but were state averages. Furthermore, transfer payments to the families of patients were mistakenly identified as costs. Both of these studies found that the day hospital alternative dominated the comparison of costs and outcomes.

As was the case with the two US studies, Dick *et al* (1985) were highly selective in the admission of patients to their trial, with the result that day hospital care presented a cost-effective alternative to hospital admission for only one-fifth of emergency admissions. In contrast to the US studies, the costing carried out in this study was comprehensive. The major limitation of the study was that attempts to compare the consequences of the treatments for the patients' social functioning and the burden of care on their families were unsuccessful.

These three studies provide some evidence of the cost-effectiveness of day-hospital as an alternative to in-patient care for patients with a range of diagnoses, but the generalisability of these results may be limited, in that each study was selective in the type of patients admitted, and that the measurement of either costs or outcomes was limited. The studies evaluated day care as an alternative to full hospital care; this leaves unanswered the question of how efficient care in day hospitals is, relative to other forms of support in the community. One study has examined this question (Linn *et al*, 1979), and it will be discussed in the final section.

Although the number of residents of psychiatric hospitals has fallen substantially in many countries in recent years, some individuals continue to enter hospital for long periods of time (Goldman *et al*, 1983). Places in the community are often not provided for the most severely disturbed individuals, who form the 'new long-stay' population of hospitals (Hyde *et al*, 1987). Although these individuals need intensive nursing care, they may not benefit from the cloistered environment of hospitals. One alternative to hospital care is care in a hostel, in close proximity to the intensive support available from a hospital. Two evaluations of such 'hostel wards' have been carried out in the UK (Wykes, 1982; Hyde *et al*, 1987; see Table 12.1). The first of these was not a controlled study, and the costing carried out was extremely limited (Wykes, 1982): the author acknowledges that the results would not generalise to other settings. The second study, carried out in Manchester, was a controlled trial. Two groups of patients were formed in matching pairs by illness duration, diagnosis, extent of psychological impairments, and remediable problem behaviour. The group to receive treatment in the hostel ward was then decided by the toss of a coin: this procedure had to be used, rather than straightforward randomisation, since the number of patients available for study was so small ($n = 22$). The authors acknowledge that the size of the study is its main weakness. However, every relevant patient produced by a catchment area of a quarter of a million over ten years was included in the study. If a larger study were to be carried out, the results of which could be generalised to other settings, then the study would have to cover a number of health districts. Both evaluations found hostel wards to be an efficient alternative to hospital wards for 'new long-stay' patients.

The efficiency of deinstitutionalisation

The decline in the resident population of psychiatric hospitals which has taken place in many countries in the last few decades has been accompanied by very little evaluation. Only one study of the costs and outcomes of discharge from psychiatric hospital exists (Linn *et al*, 1985; see Table 12.2). Another study, however, estimated the total costs of caring for individuals with schizophrenia in the community after discharge (Muller & Caton, 1983): no estimates of the costs of institutional care were made to provide a comparison. Such a comparison was made in two other studies (Cassel *et al*, 1972; Murphy & Datel, 1976): cohorts of patients discharged from psychiatric hospitals were followed into the community and the cost of care in each setting was identified, but neither study evaluated the effectiveness of hospital and community care respectively. These studies do not provide evidence on the efficiency of community care, relative to continued hospital residence. Efficiency is defined by either maximising benefit for a given cost or minimising cost for a given benefit: it is not achieved simply by cost minimisation. The least-cost alternative to in-patient care, for those with a chronic mental health problem, would be to do nothing for these individuals, but this information is not helpful in the task of developing a cost effective community care programme.

The one study which has evaluated both the costs and effectiveness of discharges from psychiatric hospitals does not provide evidence on the efficiency of deinstitutionalisation, since the alternative to hospital residence was in-patient care in a nursing home (Linn *et al*, 1985). This evaluation was based on a large (*n* = 403) RCT; nursing homes were found to be less expensive than care in psychiatric hospitals, but were also less effective.

There is next to no evidence on the cost-effectiveness of discharge from psychiatric hospitals. A study is currently being carried out on the costs and outcomes of discharging patients from Friern and Claybury Hospitals in London (Knapp, this volume), but one study cannot hope to provide answers to any more than a few questions about the efficiency of deinstitutionalisation. The paucity of evaluations of discharge versus continued hospital care may, in part, reflect the difficulty of carrying out such evaluations. On the effectiveness side, it is difficult to obtain valid evidence, since randomisation is often objected to on the ethical grounds that patients should be offered the more humanitarian community care alternative, if this is available. But the superiority of community care does not appear to be generally accepted.

TABLE 12.2
In-patient versus community care

Study	Experimental treatment (E)	Control treatment (C)	Type of patients	Type of study	Number in sample	Enumeration Outcomes	Costs	Results
Discharge versus continued hospital care								
Linn et al (1985) (USA)	Discharge to community nursing homes or units	Continued hospital stay	Male, schizophrenia or organic brain syndrome; excluded: diagnosis of cancer or life expectancy less than 1 year	RCT (1-year follow-up)	E = 245 C = 158 (89%)	Psycho-pathology, physical and mental functioning, mood, social adjustment, satisfaction	Direct treatment costs only	Nursing homes were least effective but also least expensive
Community care versus in-patient admission								
Pasamanick et al (1967) (USA)	Home care with support provided by public health nurse and drug or placebo	In-patient care	Schizophrenics with family support and not homicidal or suicidal	RCT (6–30 month follow-up)	E = 112 C = 63 (95%)	Psychiatric state, social functioning, hospitalisation	Direct costs to hospital sector only	E dominant on costs and outcomes
Coates et al (1976) (Canada)	Home treatment with some hospital care	Hospital treatment with some home care	Severely disturbed patients	Patients grouped by treatment received	150 (71%)	Symptom remission, behaviour, role performance, attitudes, satisfaction	Direct and indirect costs to health and social services; transfer payments included	Increased hospitalisation; increased costs but not outcomes

Continued

Study	Experimental	Control	Population	Design	Sample	Outcome measures	Costs	Conclusion
Mosher & Menn (1978) (USA)	Group home run by non-professional staff on a non-medical model	In-patient stay in CMHC; crisis-orientated with emphasis on use of drugs	Young (16–30 years) single schizophrenic with ≤1 in-patient admission	Allocation on space available basis (2-year follow-up)	E = 33 (89%) C = 30 (71%)	Psycho-pathology independent living, occupation, social contacts	Not identified	E dominant on costs and outcomes
Weisbrod *et al* (1980) Stein & Test (1980) (USA)	Training in community living programme	Short-term in-patient followed by after-care	All seeking admission without organic brain disorder or alcoholism (50% schizophrenic)	RCT (28-month follow-up)	E = 65 C = 65 (81% of all interviews completed)	Symptoms social functioning, employment, satisfaction, self-esteem, earnings	Direct and indirect costs to health, social, and law enforcement services; subsistence costs, family burden; capital costs	Experimental treatment produced better outcomes and higher net monetary benefit
Fenton *et al* (1979) (1982) (Canada)	Home treatment with involvement of family	In-patient stay with after-care	All seeking admission in contact with family; no violent or suicidal behaviour (40% schizophrenic)	RCT (1-year follow-up)	E = 65 (86%) C = 61 (77%)	Symptoms, role functioning	Direct and indirect treatment costs, transport costs, family burden; included transfer payments	Experimental treatment as effective and cheaper than in-patient care
Hoult *et al* (1984) (Australia)	Comprehensive community treatment	In-patient stay with after-care	All seeking admission; excluding <15 years, >65 years, organic brain disorder, alcoholism, and drug dependence	RCT (1-year follow-up)	E = 53 (88%) C = 47 (84%)	Symptoms, functioning, satisfaction, and coping	Direct and indirect costs to health and social services	E dominant on costs and outcomes

If randomisation to institutional and community care is unethical, then the ethics of the mental health policy in Scotland, where there are twice as many psychiatric in-patients relative to the size of the population than in England, must be questioned.

The costing component of such studies is not straightforward. The long-run savings from closing a hospital can be estimated from average costs, but in the short run, only certain wards can be closed, and savings cannot be estimated from average costs. In part, this is due to the point already made – that costs are related to the severity of a patient's condition; the patients discharged first are likely to be the least disturbed, thus the cost of caring for them is less than the average. Additionally, not all of the components of a hospital's costs are sensitive to the number of residents. For example, as patients are discharged, heating, lighting, and maintenance costs do not fall by much. The marginal savings from discharging patients must be calculated by allocating costs down to individual wards: these ward costs provide an estimate of the savings which can be made when a group of patients is discharged, allowing a particular ward to be closed. Similarly, the marginal, not average, costs of community care must be calculated.

Evaluation of the efficiency of deinstitutionalisation is complicated but not impossible. However, the fact that in many countries the population of psychiatric hospitals has already been substantially reduced, means that research into the efficiency of discharge to the community is of lower priority. Long-term institutionalisation has, to an extent, been replaced by a 'revolving door' policy. The primary research question now is whether support in the community can provide an efficient alternative to admission to in-patient care. Pasamanick et al (1967; see Table 12.2) evaluated care in patients' homes, with support provided by a public health nurse together with medication or placebos, as alternatives to in-patient admission. This was a good clinical trial, but the costing was very limited: the only costs identified were those to the hospital sector. In the transition from institutional to community care, the agencies providing care will change, and if the costing is not comprehensive, a shift in the burden of costs will appear as a reduction in total costs. The lower cost of community care identified by Pasamanick et al (1967) may merely reflect their narrow costing.

The study carried out by Coates et al (1976; see Table 12.2) in Canada made little improvement on the costing of the earlier study and produced less robust evidence on the effectiveness of the alternatives. This study was initially designed as an RCT, with patients being allocated to either hospital or home treatment or a combination of the two. After one year, the groups were found to be no different in the hospital stays they had experienced, and so the analysis was based on patients grouped according to the amount of both hospital and home treatment that they had actually received. This method makes it difficult to attribute outcomes to treatments, since outcomes may reflect differences in the characteristics of the patients treated.

Mosher & Menn (1978; see Table 12.2) argued that transferring in-patient care from hospitals to new institutions in the community is not consistent with the philosophy of community care. They evaluated a group home run by non-professional staff on a non-medical model with the minimum use of medication, as an alternative to in-patient care in a community mental health centre (CMHC). The evidence on the efficiency of this radical alternative to in-patient care for young schizophrenics is unfortunately limited. The study was not an RCT, and while cost figures are reported, no description is given of the items costed. The costs reported for a community care programme vary according to the range of costs identified; therefore, merely reporting cost figures with no description of the derivation of these amounts provides little information on the relative costs of the alternatives to society.

Three more recent studies provide more robust evidence on both the effectiveness and cost of community care programmes as alternatives to admission to in-patient care (Weisbrod *et al*, 1980; Fenton *et al*, 1982; Hoult *et al*, 1984; see Table 12.2). The studies carried out by Weisbrod *et al* and Hoult *et al*, in the USA and Australia respectively, both evaluated an experimental treatment which offered comprehensive support in the community, with an emphasis on training patients in basic living and social skills. In order to make the results generalisble to as many other populations as possible, few exclusion criteria were placed on entry to the study. Weisbrod *et al* excluded only those with a primary diagnosis of organic brain disorder or alcoholism, and Hoult *et al* added only drug dependency and ages of less than 16 or greater than 65 years to this exclusion list.

The most comprehensive costing component of any evaluation of mental health care was made by Weisbrod *et al* (1980): a societal perspective was taken. It is recognised that not all costs can be valued in monetary units, e.g. psychosocial burden on families, patient mortality costs, and the costs of illegal activity. In such cases, costs are simply measured in physical units, e.g. the number of families reporting physical illness as a result of the clients' condition. Other costs are even more difficult to measure, e.g., burdens on neighbours and fellow workers. Rather than omit such costs altogether, Weisbrod *et al* simply identify them. This approach of explicitly identifying all of the relevant costs and then measuring in physical units, or valuing in monetary units, as is feasible, reduces the danger of concentrating on the monetary costs of the alternatives. This is particularly important in the costing of community care, which gives a greater role to informal carers, to whom costs may not be monetary. However, the costing carried out by Hoult *et al* is less impressive; only costs to health and social services were identified, and this narrower identification of costs may explain why Hoult *et al* found community care to be less expensive than in-patient admission, while Weisbrod *et al* discovered the opposite.

A further difference between the two studies is that Weisbrod *et al* included the economic benefits of the treatments, measured by increases in labour market earnings. However, these are only part of the indirect benefits of treatment – increases in unpaid production (e.g. household, DIY) should have been included for consistency. The inclusion of labour market productivity effects has distributional implications for the results of an evaluation: programmes which benefit patients with the highest wage rates, usually used as proxies for productivity, will be favoured. Such distributional consequences should be made explicit.

In both these studies, comprehensive community care was found to be more effective than in-patient admission and after-care. The Wisconsin study also discovered that when the community programme was withdrawn after 14 months, patients' health began to deteriorate. Continuous support in the community was also one of the features Hoult *et al* identified as responsible for the success of the programme they evaluated, and there is evidence of this from many other studies (Test & Stein, 1978). Although Weisbrod *et al* found the community programme to be the most expensive alternative, the greater monetary benefits exceeded these greater costs. In both studies, support in the community was found to be more efficient than admission to in-patient care.

An RCT of a community care programme as an alternative to in-patient admission has also been carried out in Canada (Fenton *et al*, 1979, 1982); this study was more selective, including only patients in contact with their family. The community care programmes involved treatment at home by a multidisciplinary team, which, like the other two programmes evaluated, was on 24-hour call. In this programme, emphasis was placed on the involvement of the family in treatment; the support offered appears to have been less extensive and assertive than the programmes evaluated by Weisbrod *et al* (1980) and Hoult *et al* (1984). This may explain why the experimental treatment was found to be only as effective as the control. Care in the community was less costly than in-patient admission, and thus was identified as more efficient, but the costing was not as comprehensive as that carried out by Weisbrod *et al*.

These three studies, carried out, respectively, in the US, Australia, and Canada, all found support in the community to be an efficient alternative to in-patient admission followed by after-care. However, the evidence does not indicate that in-patient care can be completely replaced by community care: in every one of these studies, some patients initially allocated to care in the community were admitted to hospital at some point. The studies provide conflicting evidence about the costs of community, relative to in-patient, care: as would be expected, the evaluation which carried out the most comprehensive costing was the one which found community care to be more expensive. This underlines the point that in order to avoid regarding shifts in the burden of cost as reductions in total costs, the enumeration of the costs of community care must be as wide as possible.

Community care alternatives

There is some evidence from the studies discussed above that community care can offer an efficient alternative to hospital residence, but there remains the question of what type of care in the community is most cost-effective for individuals with particular characteristics. Unfortunately, few evaluations of alternative forms of community care have been carried out. At present, little is known about the most cost-effective way of supporting those with chronic mental health problems in the community.

An evaluation carried out in the USA assessed the efficiency of day treatment centres, in addition to drug management, for chronic schizophrenic patients discharged from hospital (Linn *et al*, 1979; see Table 12.3). The evaluation produced robust evidence on effectiveness, which showed that day treatment improved the social functioning of individuals as compared to drug management alone. Unfortunately, the only costs identified were those to hospitals and the day treatment centres; consequently, it is not possible to assess whether the provision of day treatment relieves the financial and non-financial burden on families, as would be expected.

A significant feature of this study is that it was a multicentre trial, and this makes it possible to examine the relationships between process and outcomes. Out of a total of ten centres, six showed significant improvements in delaying relapse, reducing symptoms, and changing the attitudes of patients, while four centres displayed no such benefits. Comparison of the practices of these two groups showed that the 'good' centres provided more occupational therapy and recreational activities, and generally treated patients for longer. The 'poor' centres had more professional counselling staff, used group psychotherapy more often, carried out more family counselling, and had higher patient turnover and readmission rates.

Cardin *et al* (1985; see Table 12.3) evaluated family therapy in the patient's home as an alternative to individual management of patients with schizophrenia in the community. The costing was more comprehensive than that carried out by Linn *et al* (1979), but the internal validity of the results may be questioned, given the small sample size ($n = 36$). Outcome was measured by psychopathology, social functioning, and family functioning. In order to compare the efficiency of the alternatives in terms of cost per unit of outcome, the researchers attempted to collapse the three dimensions of outcome into a single index. This was done by attributing to each subject a score of 0, 1, or 2 for each dimension, according to the initial level of impairment and the improvement experienced over time. The three scores

TABLE 12.3
Community care alternatives

Study	Experimental treatment (E)	Control treatment (C)	Type of patients	Type of study	Number in sample	Enumeration Outcomes	Enumeration Costs	Results
Linn *et al* (1979) (USA)	Day treatment plus drug management	Drug management alone	Discharged male chronic schizophrenics not previously treated in day treatment centre and no organic brain disease	RCT (2-year follow-up)	E = 80 C = 82 (85%)	Symptoms, social functioning, attitudes, readmissions	Costs incurred by hospital and day treatment centre only	All day centres improved social functioning; 6 centres improved other outcomes and reduced costs; 4 centres increased costs
Cardin *et al* (1985) (USA)	Family therapy in patients' own homes	Individual management in the community	Schizophrenics	RCT (1-year follow-up)	E = 18 (100%) C = 18 (100%)	Psycho-pathology, social functioning, family functioning	Direct and indirect costs to health and social services; law enforcement and subsistence costs	E dominant on costs and outcomes
Franklin *et al* (1987) (USA)	Case management	Existing community services (not described)	Patients with ≥2 admissions to mental hospital; not in nursing home, jail, or psychiatric in-patient facility	RCT (1-year follow-up)	E = 138 (65%) C = 126 (62%)	Readmissions, quality of life	Costs of hospital and community services	Case management increased costs but did not improve quality of life

Study	Experimental	Control	Patients	Design	Sample	Outcome measures	Cost measures	Results
Mangen et al (1983) (UK)	Therapy provided by community psychiatric nurse (CPN)	Out-patient care provided by psychiatrist	18–69 years, discharged from hospital or day care or out-patients for ≥6 months; requiring ≥6-month follow-up; majority neurotic	RCT (18-month follow-up)	E = 36 C = 35 (72%)	Symptoms, social role performance, satisfaction	Direct and indirect treatment costs to health and social services, travel costs; income loss of patients and families, family burden	Clinical and social outcomes similar; consumer satisfaction greater for CPN, which was also cheaper
Ginsberg et al (1984) (UK) Marks (1985) (UK)	Behavioural psychotherapy provided by nurse therapist	Routine treatment from general practitioner	Neurotic patients assessed as suitable for behavioural therapy	RCT (2-year follow-up)	E = 22 (48%) C = 26 (57%)	Problem and work/leisure ratings; problem related targets; fear	Costs to health service, patient, and family	E dominant on costs and outcomes

were added together for each subject to produce a summary index ranging from 0 to 6. This method of deriving an index of outcome is extremely crude and involves a number of value judgements, which were not made explicit by the authors. In the aggregation of the dimensions of outcome, equal weight was given to each dimension, and outcomes were judged to be equal if scores were equal, no matter what the composition of this score. These values, imposed by the researchers, are unlikely to be consistent with the preferences of most individuals. The imposition of values is unavoidable in the construction of an outcome index, since what is required is that one state of health be valued against another, but there is no justification for researchers simply to impose their own values. Values should reflect the preferences of a sample of psychiatrists, clients, or the population. The construction of a summary index was not even necessary in this evaluation, since family management was found to be both the most effective and the least-cost alternative.

Case management has been found to be an efficient method of organising community care for the elderly in the UK (Challis & Davies, 1986; Challis et al, 1988). A study carried out in the USA examined the efficiency of introducing case management of individuals with a chronic mental health problem living in the community (Franklin et al, 1987; see Table 12.3). The study was an RCT, with an initial sample of 417, but only 63% of this sample could be followed up for one year – a response rate which jeopardises the internal validity of the results. It was discovered that case management increased the use of both community and hospital services, but produced no improvement in quality of life. However, costs to the informal sector were not identified in the evaluation. It is possible that by increasing the use of community and hospital services, case management relieved the burden of care on the informal sector, and if this were the case, then case management is not necessarily inefficient.

Two studies carried out in the UK have examined the substitution of nurse therapists for qualified medical practitioners in the treatment of individuals suffering from chronic neuroses (Mangen et al, 1983; Ginsberg et al, 1984; see Table 12.3). One examined the use of community psychiatric nurses as an alternative to out-patient care provided by psychiatrists (Mangen et al, 1983), while the other evaluated behavioural psychotherapy provided by nurse therapists as an alternative to routine management of neuroses by general practitioners (Ginsberg et al, 1984). Both studies were based on an RCT, but small sample sizes and relatively high drop-out rates mean that the results may not have internal validity. In the study by Ginsberg et al, there were substantial differences between the two groups in use of resources, prior to entry to the study, while in both, atypical use of services by a few patients generated differences in total costs between the groups. Both studies found nurse therapists to be an efficient alternative to treatment by medical practitioners. The results of these two studies indicate some scope for using nurses to substitute for medical and psychiatric specialists in helping sufferers overcome the problems of neurotic behaviour, but the studies are very specific to the situations in which they were operated, and therefore difficult to generalise into common practice. The further problems of giving nurses special training for specific conditions, and the effect this might have on their other duties or the organisation of the profession, have not been examined.

Conclusion

There is a lack of evidence on the efficiency of community care for those with a chronic mental health problem. A relatively small number of evaluations have been carried out, and many are deficient in one or more respects. There is some evidence that day hospitals provide an efficient alternative to in-patient care (Washburn *et al*, 1976; Endicott *et al*, 1978; Dick *et al*, 1985). But these results were obtained for particular types of individuals, and in two of the studies the costing was very narrow, while in the other one, important dimensions of outcome could not be measured adequately.

Comprehensive programmes of support in the community have been shown to be more efficient than in-patient admissions for people with a wide range of diagnoses (Weisbrod *et al*, 1980; Fenton *et al*, 1982; Hoult *et al*, 1984), but three studies cannot provide answers to all of the questions about the efficiency of community care as an alternative to hospital residence. In an effort to make the results generalisable, the authors of these studies were not particularly selective in admitting patients to the trials. But in each case, the results were presented for the 'average individual'; in fact, few individuals look like the average. If one is to determine the applicability of the results of an evaluation to a particular individual, then disaggregated results are required (Knapp, 1987). A further point about the generalisability of the results of these studies is that, in all three evaluated model programmes, their effectiveness results may, in part, derive from the enthusiasm of staff for such programmes, and this would not necessarily be experienced in other settings (Freedman & Moran, 1984).

These three studies provide little information on the relationships between the processes of community care and outcomes. There is some evidence that, to be effective, care in the community should be comprehensive, assertive, and continuous; in order to gather more evidence on what particular features of community care are most effective, a large number of studies based on the same methods, but evaluating slightly different programmes of support, would have to be carried out. Currently, only a handful of evaluations of alternative types of community care have been completed. Day treatment of people with schizophrenia was found to be more efficient than drug management alone (Linn *et al*, 1979), and family therapy more efficient than individual management in the community (Cardin *et al*, 1985). Case management was found to be an inefficient method of organising community care (Franklin *et al*, 1987), but the substitution of nurse therapists for general practitioners and psychiatrists in the treatment of neuroses was found to be efficient (Ginsberg *et al*, 1984; Mangen *et al*, 1983). However, each of these studies has at least one limitation which makes it difficult to generalise the results.

The efficiency of many varieties of community care remains unevaluated. For example, nothing is known about the efficiency of providing day care through community mental health centres as an alternative to day hospitals; whether the location of care in primary care settings would be more efficient than in specialist institutions is not known; the efficiency of 24-hour crisis teams is unevaluated; and the efficiency of alternative types of residential provision, e.g. group homes, family homes, and supported landlord or landlady schemes, is also unknown. Similarly, nothing is known of the efficiency of alternative types of employment training. Much work remains to be done before the most efficient programme of community support for individuals with particular characteristics can be identified.

There is also room for improvement in the methods of the evaluations. On the costing side, the main point is that efficiency should be assessed from a societal perspective: it is not sufficient to identify the costs of community care to health and other social services – the costs to the voluntary and informal sectors are just as relevant. Without comprehensive costing, community care can be made to look cheap, merely as a result of shifting the burden of care away from the hospital sector. In order to avoid underestimation of the costs of community care, the approach of Weisbrod *et al* (1980) is recommended: all costs should be explicitly identified, even if they cannot all be measured in monetary units.

Most studies have relied on average costs to estimate the costs of community and institutional care, but since in most cases the alternatives have been the expansion of the former and contraction of the latter, it is marginal, not average, costs which should be used. Most studies have excluded capital costs from the appraisal: this is a serious omission in evaluations of community versus institutional care – alternatives which have vastly different capital requirements.

The lack of information about the efficiency of alternative programmes of care for those with a chronic mental health problem makes it impossible to identify alternatives which offer greater benefits than those generated from the current deployment of resources. Such a situation is wasteful of resources: the available resources are not being used to maximise the quality of life of clients.

Acknowledgements

I would like to acknowledge the financial support of the Economic and Social Research Council and to thank Alan Maynard, Alan Shiell, and Ken Wright for comments on an earlier draft. I accept full responsibility for any remaining errors.

References

CARDIN, V. A., McGILL, C. W. & FALLOON, I. R. H. (1985) Economic analysis: costs, benefits and effectiveness. In *Family Management of Schizophrenia: A Study of Clinical, Social and Economic Benefits*, (eds I. R. H. Falloon *et al*), pp. 115–123. Baltimore, MD: Johns Hopkins University Press.

CASSELL, W. A., SMITH, C. N., GRUNBERG, F., *et al* (1972) Comparing costs of hospital and community care. *Hospital and Community Psychiatry*, **23**, 197–200.

CHALLIS, D. & DAVIES, B. (1986) *Case Management in Community Care*. Aldershot: Gower.

——, CHESSUM, R., CHESTERMAN, J., *et al* (1988) Community care for the frail elderly: an urban experience. *British Journal of Social Work* (suppl.), 13–42.

COATES, D. B., KENDALL, L. M., MACURDY, E. A., *et al* (1976) Evaluating hospital and home treatment of psychiatric patients. A one-year follow-up. *Canada's Mental Health*, **24**, 28–32.

DICK, P., CAMERON, L., COHEN, D., *et al* (1985) Day and full-time psychiatric treatment: a controlled comparison. *British Journal of Psychiatry*, **147**, 246–250.

ENDICOTT, J., HERZ, M. & GIBBON, M. (1978) Brief versus standard hospitalisation: the differential costs. *American Journal of Psychiatry*, **135**, 707–712.

FENTON, F. R., TESSIER, L. & STRUENING, E. L. (1979) A comparative trial of home and hospital psychiatric care. *Archives of General Psychiatry*, **36**, 1073–1079.

——, ——, ——, *et al* (1982) *Home and Hospital Psychiatric Treatment*. London: Croom Helm.

FRANKLIN, J. L., SOLOVITZ, B., MASON, M., *et al* (1987) An evaluation of case management. *American Journal of Public Health*, **77**, 674–678.

FREEDMAN, R. I. & MORAN, A. (1984) Wanderers in a promised land: the chronically mentally ill and deinstitutionalisation. *Medical Care*, **22**(suppl. 12).

GINSBERG, G., MARKS, I. & WATERS, H. (1984) Cost-benefit analysis of a controlled trial of nurse therapy for neuroses in primary care. *Psychological Medicine*, **14**, 683–690.

GLICK, I., HARGREAVES, A. & GOLDFIELD, M. D. (1974) Short versus long hospitalisation: a prospective controlled study. *Archives of General Psychiatry*, **30**, 363–369.

GOLDMAN, H., MORRISEY, J. & BACHRACH, L. (1983) Deinstitutionalisation in international perspective. *International Journal of Mental Health*, **11**, 153–165.

HÄFNER, H. & AN DER HEIDEN, W. (1989) Effectiveness and cost of community care for schizophrenic patients. *Hospital and Community Psychiatry*, **40**, 59–63.

HOULT, J., ROSEN, A. & REYNOLDS, I. (1984) Community orientated treatment compared to psychiatric hospital orientated treatment. *Social Science and Medicine*, **18**, 1005–1010.

HYDE, C., BRIDGES, K., GOLDBERG, D., *et al* (1987) The evaluation of a hostel ward, a controlled study using modified cost-benefit analysis. *British Journal of Psychiatry*, **151**, 805–812.

JONES, R. & GOLDBERG, D. (1980) The costs and benefits of psychiatric care. In *The Social Consequences of Psychiatric Illness*, (eds L. Robins, P. Clayton & J. K. Wing), pp. 55–70. New York: Brunner/Mazel.

——, —— & HUGHES, B. (1980) A comparison of two different services treating schizophrenia, cost-benefit approach. *Psychological Medicine*, **10**, 493–505.

KNAPP, M. (1987) *Economic Barriers to Innovation in Mental Health Care: Community Care in the UK*. Discussion Paper no. 541/2, Personal Social Services Research Unit, University of Kent at Canterbury.

—— (1991) The direct costs of the community care of chronically mentally ill people. In *Evaluation of Comprehensive Care of the Mentally Ill* (eds H. Freeman & J. Henderson), pp. 142–173. London: Gaskell.

LEVENSON, A. J., LORD, C. J., SERMAS, C. E., *et al* (1977) Acute schizophrenia: an efficacious out-patient treatment approach as an alternative to full-time hospitalisation. *Diseases of the Nervous System*, 242–245.

LINN, M. W., CAFFEY, E. G., KLETT, J., *et al* (1979) Day treatment and psychotropic drugs in the aftercare of schizophrenic patients. *Archives of General Psychiatry*, **36**, 1055–1066.

——, GUREL, L., WILLFORD, W. U., *et al* (1985) Nursing home care as an alternative to psychiatric hospitalisation. *Archives of General Psychiatry*, **42**, 544–551.

MANGEN, S. P., PAYKEL, E. S., GRIFFITH, J. H., *et al* (1983) Cost-effectiveness of community psychiatric nurse or out-patient psychiatrist care of neurotic patients. *Psychological Medicine*, **13**, 407–416.

MARKS, I. (1985) Controlled trial of psychiatric nurse therapists in primary care. *British Medical Journal*, **290**, 1181–1184.

MOSHER, L. R. & MENN, A. Z. (1978) Community residential treatment for schizophrenia: two-year follow-up. *Hospital and Community Psychiatry*, **29**, 715–723.

MULLER, C. F. & CATON, C. L. M. (1983) Economic costs of schizophrenia: a post-discharge study. *Medical Care*, **21**, 92–103.

MURPHY, J. G. & DATEL, W. E. (1976) A cost-benefit analysis of community versus institutional living. *Hospital and Community Psychiatry*, **27**, 165–170.

PASAMANICK, B., SCARPITTI, F. & DINITZ, S. (1967) *Schizophrenics in the Community: An Experimental Study in the Prevention of Hospitalisation.* New York: Appleton-Century-Crofts.

SOUTHAMPTON PSYCHIATRIC CASE REGISTER (1983) Stein, L. I. & Test, M. A. (1980) Alternative to mental hospital treatment. *Archives of General Psychiatry*, **37**, 392–397.

TEST, M. A. & STEIN, L. I. (1978) Community treatment of the chronic patient: research overview. *Schizophrenia Bulletin*, **4**, 350–364.

WASHBURN, S., VANNICELLI, M., LONGABAUGH, R., *et al* (1976) A controlled comparison of psychiatric day treatment and in-patient hospitalisation. *Journal of Consulting and Clinical Psychology*, **44**, 665–675.

WEISBROD, B. A., TEST, M. A. & STEIN, L. I. (1980) An alternative to mental hospital treatment. II: Economic benefit-cost analysis. *Archives of General Practice*, **37**, 400–405.

WYKES, T. (1982) A hostel-ward for 'new' long-stay patients: an evaluative study of a ward in a house. In *Long-term Community Care: Experience in a London Borough. Psychological Medicine, monograph suppl. 2*, (ed. J. K. Wing). Cambridge: Cambridge University Press.

13 National reports

France: **ROGER AMIEL**

French public psychiatry has been comprehensive for almost 40 years. In 1987, the country was divided into 800 Sectors for general psychiatry and 298 for child and adolescent psychiatry; in general psychiatry, the average catchment population was 71 600. One-third of these Sectors are attached to a general and not to a psychiatric hospital; the average number of beds available per Sector is 106. On one day (15 December 1985), there was an average of 89 patients per Sector in hospital. In 1987, each Sector saw an average of 937 new patients: half of these were seen as out-patients, a quarter as hospital referrals, and the remainder had both in-patient and out-patient care. In recent years, the number of admissions has been increasing.

The first administrative circular of March 1960 established the policy of Sectorisation, with a *Chef de Service*, but it was not until 1985 that the financial problems were resolved. Since then, the activities of the whole Sector, including prevention, have been financed by Social Security. Within each Sector, there are contacts with all the private charities or voluntary organisations with which the service can work, and they also receive some financial support.

The Ninth Health Plan, ending in 1990, has proposed the closure or conversion of 40 000 beds out of the 110 000 which existed in 1981; up to the end of 1989, 20 000 had been closed. However, the budgets of these Sectors remained the same, even if beds were closed; the money can be used for out-patient facilities or other services. For many years, some Sectors have been undertaking local studies to evaluate what they are doing, but nothing of that sort is possible on a very large scale.

The number of psychotic patients under care is no greater than it was 20 years ago, but there are many more identified neurotic and psychosomatic cases. Patients can go either to their GPs about these conditions (particularly for anxiety problems), or directly to psychiatrists.

197

Allowing for inflation, there is approximately the same amount of money ('global budget') available each year. Six months before the commencement of the year, this is discussed with representatives of the Ministry of Health and of the Social Security System. Discussions are then held between the heads of the various services within the Sector, as to how the money should be utilised. For instance, there might be a proposal for a sheltered flat, or to replace a post for a psychiatrist by an extra nurse for out-patients or extra social workers. There is an administrative requirement to specify how the money has been spent and to evaluate the results.

Greece: NICOLAS ZACHARIADIS

Until very recently, mental health care in Greece was largely based on psychiatric hospitals, of which there are ten in the country. Owing to the facts that a sectorisation policy has not yet reached an adequate level of functioning and that hospital catchment areas are still ill-defined, continuity of care after discharge is not established, and the 'revolving door' phenomenon is consequently common.

However, out of 8149 patients who were resident in public psychiatric hospitals, according to a one-day census in 1982, only 6377 were still recorded in a similar census in 1990; beds in private psychiatric clinics declined by nearly 800 within the same period.

These findings might be related to the fact that within the 12 mental health regions into which the country has been divided, just over 100 primary and secondary care units are now functioning, and although their distribution is characterised by a high density in urban areas and a scarcity in the provinces, they must contribute to keeping patients out of hospital by providing alternative care.

In a questionnaire sent to 24 consultant psychiatrists working in public psychiatric hospitals, which focused on the parameters that might have influenced the above-mentioned reduction of psychiatric in-patients between 1982 and 1989 and the shift towards extramural care, the modern training of psychiatrists ranked first in priority, and the more detailed screening of patients for hospital admission second. Mortality among hospital residents was considered to be even less significant.

The Netherlands: DURK WIERSMA

In the Netherlands, the general policy on mental health care is focused on shortening stay in mental hospitals and on the resettlement of long-stay patients in sheltered accommodation. It was planned that about 2000 long-stay patients should be transferred to sheltered accommodation by 1990, together with more coordination of services, geographical dispersal of hospital facilities, and strengthening of extramural services.

During the 1980s, the overall health and mental health budgets ceased to grow, even showing a little decrease. The Government is now more focused on a policy of deregulation, preferring to stand back from central planning and central prescription. Functional regionalisation has become an important principle; there is no longer any requirement to plan for institutions, but more for functions and for programmes of care and treatment aimed at sections of each defined population – elderly, adult, schizophrenic, etc. Attention will be diverted from institutions to programmes for health care, and the key word in this process of restructuring is 'substitution', meaning a shift from care to prevention; from full-time to partial hospitalisation and day care; from long-term to short-term treatment; and, last but not least, from the expensive to the less expensive.

During the 1980s, there was about a 2% decrease in the number of beds in mental hospitals (which number 48). Psychiatric departments in general hospitals have decreased in size further, although their actual total is only 2400 beds; however, the number of psychogeriatric places has shown a large increase to 23 000. Sheltered living accommodation in the community has increased by only 10% in the last ten years. Community mental health centres employ only a very small proportion of the personnel in mental health care, but they have increased in number by 36%. Over the last three years, a stable 83% of expenditure has gone to the intramural sector, 4–5% to part-time care (sheltered accommodation), and 12% to extramural care; this has become a fairly fixed ratio. The total mental health budget is about 15% of total health costs; for 1990, an increase of US $12 million was budgeted for, of which only $2.5 million (21%) was allocated to extramural care.

Several projects focusing on the shift from intramural to extramural care are now in progress. One of them is the substitution project in Drenthe, in which the feasibility of day treatment with community care, as an alternative to conventional 24-hour mental hospital care, is being tested in a randomised experiment: it has already been shown that 38% of an unselected severely ill population can be satisfactorily treated in a day programme. Other projects (Maastricht, Utrecht) with experimental research designs are evaluating the effects of a Social Psychiatric Service Centre and of day treatment, as substitutes for ordinary hospital care. In addition, new developments with respect to patients' rights, improvement of housing conditions, day activities centres, and psychiatric rehabilitation are in progress in various parts of the Netherlands.

Portugal: JOSÉ CALDAS DE ALMEIDA

Portugal is a small country consisting of three regions, each with a large city. In the 1960s, the mental health service consisted of only two mental hospitals in each of these three cities, but, in 1963, a new Mental Health Law was approved, very much influenced by the sectorisation policy in France. This established the division of the country into Sectors, with a mental health service in each. During the 1960s and 1970s, 18 mental health centres were created; these have the responsibility for all psychiatric care of a defined population, including the in-patient facilities.

At the same time, centres for the treatment of children and of drug addiction were created in each of the three large cities. In the mental hospitals, the most important change was a significant decrease in the number of resident patients. A very important measure, in 1984, was the integration of all mental health services, including mental hospitals, into the General Directorate of Primary Health Care. This was shortly after the decision that the basis for all health systems was to be a network of health centres, and the key worker of these health systems was to be the general practitioner.

In 1985, the mental health programme presented by the Director of Mental Health Services was approved, and the main goals established were the development of community services and the integration of mental health care and rehabilitation into primary health care. First, however, the psychiatric catchment areas were redefined to correspond with the areas of the health centres, so that it would be possible for the mental health teams to work together with the health centre teams.

A new model of financing projects was implemented, and the priorities chosen were those projects that encouraged working with GPs and helped towards the creation of community programmes. Many mental health staff began to work with family doctors, mainly using the catchment area model. In 1988, the Ministry of Health decided to reinforce the implementation of this programme, as a contribution towards solving three main problems.

Firstly, new services had to be created in the three large cities, which still had only mental hospitals. Secondly, when the budget and staff of the mental hospitals were compared with those in the mental health centres, the hospitals were seen to be responsible for 40% of the population and the centres for almost 60%. Yet 80% of the budget remains concentrated on the old mental hospitals; therefore, we have the problem of how to transfer the resources to the new kind of services. Thirdly, approval was given to the plan for reorganising the mental health services, and the following guidelines were considered fundamental in this process:

(a) *Sectorisation*, in which the care system is organised according to defined catchment areas with about 75 000 inhabitants; these will be the responsibility of the multidisciplinary teams in mental health centres.
(b) *Continuity of care*, which implies that patients are always dealt with by the same team within the various levels of care in order to ensure

continuity of the therapeutic relationship, a continuity which is fundamental in mental health.

(c) *Technical and administrative autonomy of the mental health services*, which is essential to ensure continuity of care and the specificity of the mental health care team.

(d) *Interrelationship between mental health and the remaining health structures*, i.e. health centres and general hospitals.

(e) *The development of community-based care*, which should progressively replace that provided in large psychiatric hospitals.

It is known that most psychiatric patients are dealt with, sometimes exclusively, by general practitioners. It is also known that the GP is usually able to help with greater efficacy if he is supported by a mental health team. If we add the fact that measures for promoting mental health necessarily include cooperation between the mental health team and the health centre team, it becomes clear why the encouragement of this relationship represents a priority. The same could be said about the interrelationship with the general hospital, which can be developed mainly at three levels: through the implementation of psychiatric in-patient services; through the integration of psychiatrists into the emergency services; and through the development of liaison psychiatry facilities, to give support to the different services of general hospitals.

A team or organisation now exists in each sector that must articulate with the health centres and GPs, and this in turn must become integrated with the general hospital. These teams are responsible for all the care, treatment, preventive work, and rehabilitation of the mentally ill. The objective is the full development of a mental health service in all regions (including in-patient units in the general hospital of the area), e.g. the development of an information system, professional training, etc.

From the point of view of evaluation, we have a case register, in the area of Porto, and it was planned to extend this to the whole country during 1991. There are also some studies, mainly of integration with primary health care, although these are not sophisticated in design. The results from teams that have worked together with primary health care show that hospital admissions have decreased by about 30%, whereas the number of patients that psychiatrists see has increased. This means that the mental health teams are receiving more referrals, but they see mainly first consultations, whereas the rest are mainly seen by the GPs.

In a fairly short time 7000 young GPs have been recruited, and a mandatory period of experience in mental health has been included in their overall training. Finally, it would be worthwhile mentioning that, in the 1970s, psychiatric units in general hospitals were restricted to three university departments. However, this situation has changed since the beginning of the 1980s, when it was decided to create psychiatric units in all new general hospitals.

Spain: CARLOS ARTUNDO PURROY

Navarre is a fairly small region in northeast Spain, with half a million inhabitants. It has eight Mental Health Sectors and 51 Health Zones, each Mental Health Sector having around 60 000 inhabitants.

In 1986, there was a regional reorganisation, embodied in a Mental Health Plan, involving the process of change and transformation of the old psychiatric hospital. There is one Mental Health Manager and two Directors, each Director having responsibility for one zone of four community health centres. Each mental health centre is to be integrated into the primary health care centre, i.e. physically into the same building. There are two day hospitals for the region, and two in-patient wards of 27 and 30 beds that are situated in the general hospital. Each team at a community health centre is responsible for all mental health problems in the Sector, and it consists of two psychiatrists, two psychologists, two nurses, one social worker, and one administrative worker. There are two specialised rehabilitation units each with 12 beds, and the staff prefer that, before being discharged into the community, patients have at least six months' intensive rehabilitation. Between 1987 and 1989, out of 701 long-stay patients, 47 (all very old) have died in hospital, 65 have been discharged to old people's residences of the Social Services, 27 to supervised flats, and eight to homes. All patients are being followed up by the same team. All mental health professionals are taking part in discussions on the information system; records of the services as well as of individual patients are cumulative, related to the geographical and the population area of each of the services.

Evaluation of the reform includes initial information on the management of the services, including studies of all drug addicts in contact with services, young psychotics, and other community offenders. The information system monitors continuity of care, and the relationship with primary care. Whereas in 1987 only 18% of the patients seen by psychiatrists were referred by their GPs, two years later 50% of all patients come from the primary health care professionals.

Of the 17 regions in Spain, three or four have made progress along the same lines as Navarre.

The information system

The information system was set up in January 1987, based in the Community Services Network; it replaced a previous system in the psychiatric hospital, which collected data from the various units there. At first, seven out of the eight mental health centres participated in the process, but later in the year, the Estella Centre was also incorporated into it. A special register was set up for the two day hospitals and for the day centre for drug addiction; the activities of Social Services for drug addicts were also incorporated. Another special register collects information about chronic patients who are discharged from the psychiatric hospital; it records where they are living and which MHC is responsible for their psychiatric care.

The system is a longitudinal register, recording all the contacts made by patients with designated services; the denominator consists of the known population of the catchment area, which has defined geographical limits. Information is stored in cumulative form, so that follow-up studies are possible; it is comprehensive, including all age groups and diagnoses. All professional staff working in the network (and particularly those in the MHCs) complete a form every day, recording all their contacts with patients. This integrated network provides the basis for planning services for the whole region.

Thus, the information system covers eight MHCs, two day hospitals, a day centre for drug addiction, and two psychiatric units in hospitals. It collects data on all contacts of patients with MHCs every day, and on admission and discharges at day hospitals. Its uses may be divided into several categories:

(a) *Clinical* – improving the efficiency of the service and continuity of care; evaluating particular forms of service (e.g. urgent attendance at an MHC or day hospital); providing information on the needs of particular groups of patients for which services could be developed; following-up specific diagnostic groups.

(b) *Planning and evaluation* – providing statistical and epidemiological information as a basis for the distribution of resources; monitoring the degree of achievement of specific objectives and the application of corrective measures; comparative evaluation of different methods of treatment or care.

(c) *Investigation* – obtaining specific samples of patients for particular studies; providing a database for epidemiological research.

The limitations of information systems such as this one are well known – primarily that they can record only administrative morbidity, as recorded by specific services, and not 'total' morbidity in the community served.

Index

compiled by STANLEY THORLEY

accessibility: items in psychiatric services
132
assertive behaviour encouraged in therapy
110
assessment issues 82–85
data management and analysis 85
effectiveness of services 3–5 & Fig. 1.2
Environmental Index (EI) 84
Patient Attitude Questionnaire (PAQ) 84
Personal Data and Psychiatric History
schedule (PDPH) 83
Physical Health Index (PHI) 83
Present State Examination (PSE) 83
Social Behaviour Schedule (SBS) 83–84
Social Network Schedule (SNS) 84
use of community facilities 84–85
Australia
Melbourne 'Psychopolis' 69
Quality Assurance Project 134

Better services for the Mentally Ill (1975) 121

Camberwell: asylum needs 49
Canada: effectiveness of alternatives 184
Table 12.2, 186–187
'Care in the community' programme
comprehensive costing 150–151 &
Table 11.1
outcomes 165–167
care programmes 50–51
Caring for People 51
case management 190 Table 12.3, 191
changes in the care system: evaluation
68–78
client characteristics
Client Service Receipt Interview
(CSRI) 150
costs and outcomes 167–169 & Table
11.7

clinical psychologists: role in primary care
121–122
'clubhouse' models 49–50, 54
cognitive–behavioural approaches to
training
information processing models 106
Integrated Psychological Treatment
Programme (IPT) 107
problem-solving 105–106
self-instruction 106
'training packages' or 'modules' 105
Commission of the European Communities
(CEC) ix–x, xi
community care
alternatives 189–193 & Table 12.3
case management 190 Table 12.3,
192
drug management alone 189–190
Table 12.3
family therapy 189–190 Table 12.3
nurse therapists 191 Table 12.3,
192–193
cost–effectiveness 174–196
criteria of successful placement 91–92
hospital comparisons 167
monitoring and evaluation 3
Italy 30–44
reforms 51
reprovision costs: Friern/Claybury
159–162 & Tables 11.3–11.5
Community Care – Agenda for Action 51, 55
Community Psychiatric Nurses (CPNs)
120–121
Concerted Action Committee Health
Service Research (COMAC-HSR) xi,
xiii
costs
client characteristics and outcomes
167–169 & Table 11.7

community care 142–173
four rules for research 144–145
  comprehensive measurement 145–151
  cost variations 151–156
  like with like comparisons 157–164
  merging costs with outcomes 164–170
indicators of appropriate care 14–15 &
    Fig. 1.6
other influences 169–170
creaming off: Friern/Claybury reprovision
    88–89 & Table 2

day hospitals 179 Table 12.1, 181–182
deinstitutionalisation
  contributory factors 24–25
  efficiency 183–189 & Table 12.2
  evaluation 58 & Fig. 5.1
  implications for professionals 25–26
  institutional standards 25
  some models 69
  transition to the community 46–48
Denmark: 'good hospital standards' 25
design
  community placement trials 79–80 &
      Fig. 7.1, 92–96
  evaluative studies 8, 10–12 & Fig. 1.3
domiciliary visits: rates 132–133 & Fig.
    10.1
Douglas House study 47–48
'dowries' or 'bounties': money transfers
    tied to bed closures 154–156, 158
drug management alone 189–190 Table
    12.3

economic study: long stay patients in
    community care 86–87
economic valuations: framework 175–176
Environmental Index (EI) 84
Europe
  Community Comprehensive Mental
      Health Service 133
  reviews of mental health policy 61–63
evaluations
  effectiveness of wider social networks
      58–60 & Fig. 5.2
  future international studies 137–138
  issues 73–74
  methodology 1–23
    community mental health services 3
    levels 1
    national health systems 1–3 & Fig.
        1.1 & Tab. 1.1
    top–down and bottom–up approaches
        19
extrapolations: costs to full populations
    162–164 & Table 11.6

family therapy 189–190 Table 12.3
Finland: schizophrenia follow–up 94
fragmentation of psychiatric services 123
framework of economic valuations
    175–176
France
  community networks: *secteurs* 66–67
  national report 197–198
Friern/Claybury reprovision 46–47
  accumulation of new long–stay patients
      87–88 & Table 7.1
  costs 159–162 & Tables 11.3–11.5
  creaming off 88–89 & Table 2
future developments 50–52, 137–138

generalisations: applications of training to
    real life situations 107–108
Georgia: Open door in Savannah 54
Greece
  national report 198
  Thessalonika community care 54
Griffiths report: *Community care – Agenda for
    Action* 51, 54

halfway houses 54
Hawthorne effect 11 & Fig. 1.5, 70–71
Health Service evaluation 127–128 &
    Table 1
"hive system" 117
homelessness 48–49
hospital–based alternatives 176–183 &
    Table 12.1
  day hospitals 179 Table 12.1, 181–182
  hostel wards 179 Table 12.1, 182
    Douglas House 47–48
  out–patient clinics 177–178 Table 12.1,
      180
  psychiatric units in general hospitals
      176–177 Table 1
hospitalisation, partial 73–74

indicators
  direct costs 14–15 & Fig. 1.6
  mental health care 6–8 & Fig. 1.3, 9
      Fig. 1.4
  output 6–8 & Fig. 1
  resources 130
  social isolation 18
Ireland: psychiatric practice 125
Italy
  costs 127–129 & Tables 10.1–10.2
  Cremona and Mantua catchment areas:
      comparison 122
  law 180 30–31, 39
  Lombardy: *converzionati* 38, 39

Lombardy
  community care services 31–32 &
      Fig. 3.1, 33 Table 3.2, 39–40
  domiciliary visits 132–133 & Fig. 10.1
  Milan area 31–40 & Fig. 3.1 & Tables
      3.1–3.7
  hospital psychiatric units 36–38 &
      Table 3.6
  intermediate residential facilities
      38–39 & Table 3.7
  out–patient services 31–36 & Tables
      1–5
Sardinia and Tuscany: mental health
      service costs 127–129 & Tables
      10.1–10.2
South Verona 40–43
  retrospective follow–up of
      schizophrenic patients 41–42
Venice and Piedmont: community
      services 63

Japan: expansion of mental hospital
      population 79
Jarman index 18, 87–88 & Table 7.1

like with like comparisons 157–164
London workshop (1989) xii, xiii
long–stay patients
  placement benefits? 79–96
  economic study 86–87
  methods and study instruments 94–96
  new accumulations 87–88 & Table 7.1
  planning a study 92–94
  sociological study 85–86

Madison training in community living
      programme 147
management components 130
Manchester
  comparisons between district general and
      area mental hospitals 176
  psychiatric primary care clinics 118
Mangen, Steen. *Mental Health Care in the
      European Community* ix
marginal opportunity costs 149, 155–156
Massachusetts
  cost–effectiveness of day hospitals
      181–182
  day–hospital–inn programme 61, 69
Maudsley daily living programme 147
mental disability: criteria 98
mental health care
  assessment of effectiveness of services
      3–4 & Fig. 1.2
  comparison of programmes 14–15 &
      Fig. 1.9

design of studies 8–14 & Fig. 1.5,
      19–21
  evaluation 26–28
  goals 4, 6, 19–21
  output indicators 6–8 & Fig. 1.3, 9
      Fig. 1.4
*Mental Health Care in the European
      Community*. Steen Mangen ix
mental health professionals 25–26
merging costs with outcomes 164–170
methodology of evaluative studies 1–23

national reports 197–203
  France 197–198
  Greece 198
  Netherlands 198–199
  Portugal 199–201
  Spain 201–203
naturalistic approaches 12–14, 20
needs
  asylum 49–50
  concept 21–22
  measurement 137
Netherlands
  national report 198–199
  substitution of hospital beds 71–73
New York
  cost–effectiveness of day hospitals
      181–182
  Fountain House 49–50, 54
NHS reforms 51–52
Nottingham
  domiciliary visits 132
  psychiatrists in general practice 122
nurse therapists 191 Table 12.3, 192–193

out–patient clinics 177–178 Table 12.1,
      180
outcome evaluation 134–137
  measurement of needs 137
  satisfaction 136–137
  self–evaluation 135
  sentinel events 136
  variables 60–61

Patient Attitude Questionnaire (PAQ) 84
performance and accessibility 131–133 &
      Fig. 10.1
Personal Data and Psychiatric History
      schedule (PDPH) 83
Personal Social Services Research Unit
      (PSSRU) study 47
  evaluation of 'Care in the community
      programme' 150–151 Table 11.1,
      159, 165
Physical Health Index (PHI) 83

Portugal: national report   199–201
predictions, cost   160–162 & Tables
    11.4–11.5
Present State Examination (PSE)   83
primary care: integration of mental health
    services   115–126
process evaluation   133–134
process or outcome approaches   127–141
programme variation   58–59 & Fig. 5.2
psychiatric units in general hospitals
    176–177 Table 12.1
psychiatrists in primary care settings
    116–117, 126
  consultation models   118–120 & Table
    9.1
  liaison attachment models   118
  shifted out–patient models   118–120 &
    Table 9.1

Quality assurance in mental health
    138–140 Appendix
'quality of life'   19–20, 27–28
quasi-experimental approaches   12, 20
  differences from randomised control
    (RCT)   157

randomised control trials (RCT)   152–153,
    157
  day hospitals   181
Report on a study of community care (1981)
    121
resources   129–130
  indicators   130
'rights' of society (carers and providers)
    110
Royal College of Psychiatrists
  guidelines on discharge procedures   51
  joint conference with Department of
    Health (1986): "ideal service"   115
'rubbishing phase'   143

Salford: domiciliary visits   132
satisfaction: patients and relatives
    136–137
schizophrenia
  community care in West Germany   62
  comparisons between district general and
    area mental hospitals   176
  Finnish follow–up   94
  gestalt of social network   66
  social skills training   104–107
  South Verona follow–up study   41–42

WHO Pilot Areas study   68
Scotland: psychiatrists associated with
    primary care   115
sentinel events: negative and positive   136
services: results of research and
    experience   45–56
  current situation   45
Social Behaviour Schedule (SBS)   83–84
social competence   97–114
Social Network Schedule (SNS)   84
social networks: effectiveness   57–67
social security payments   148, 150
social skills   99–100
  cognitive–behavioural approaches
    105–107
  training (SST)   101–103
    general outcome   103–105
sociological study: long stay patients in
    community care   85–86
Spain: national report   201–203
'substitution models': Netherlands   71–73

Team for the Assessment of Psychiatric
    Services (TAPS)
  community reprovision costs:
    Friern/Claybury   86–87, 159–162 &
    Tables 11.3–11.5
  design issues   79–82 & Fig. 7.1
  preliminary findings   89–90
thresholds or standards   139
top–down and bottom–up approaches   19
'transfer payments'   148
transition to the community *see*
    deinstitutionalisation
treatment strategies: effectiveness   24–29

UK survey: current situation   45

variations, cost   151–156
  hospitals   154–156 & Table 11. 2

West Germany: community care for
    schizophrenics   62
Wisconsin: 'Training in Community
    Living'   69
Worcester Development Project   49, 69
Working for Patients   51
World Health Organization (WHO)
  effectiveness in planning   57
  importance of primary care   115–116
  Pilot Areas study   68
'worried well': drift of resources   46, 53, 54